The
GOODBYE
BACK PAIN
Handbook

The
GOODBYE
BACK PAIN
Handbook

James A. Peterson and James Wheeler

MASTERS PRESS

Published by Masters Press, 5025 28th Street, S.E,
Grand Rapids, Michigan 49506

This book is not intended to be a substitute for medical care.
Anyone suffering from back problems should, of course, consult
a physician. Neither the authors nor the publisher assumes
responsibility for the reader's treatment.

The views expressed herein are those of the authors and do not
purport to reflect the position of the United States Military
Academy, the Department of the Army or the Department of
Defense.

Library of Congress Cataloging-in-Publication Data

Peterson, James A., 1943–
    The goodbye back pain handbook: how to treat and
    prevent back pain / James A. Peterson and James Wheeler.
       p. cm.
    ISBN 0-940279-20-7
    1. Backache — Popular works. I. Wheeler, James. 1950– .
II. Title.
RD771.B217P47 1988   88-29564
617'.56 — dc19   CIP

DEDICATION

To the Corps of Cadets and the staff and faculty of the United States Military Academy, whose quality and zest for life motivated us to develop a safer, more effective means of treating back pain.

CONTENTS

ACKNOWLEDGMENTS

Almost every book endeavor is the final product of the collective contributions of several individuals. Ours is no different. Colonel Al Rushatz and Dr. William J. Penny have been a valuable source of friendship and sound advice. Elaine Pettine, Jane Reddington and Susan Rothenbusch provided superb typing assistance. We also owe a tremendous debt of gratitude to our wives, Sandee Wheeler and Sue Peterson, for their support, understanding and patience during this project.

We would also like to express our appreciation to the many back patients we've treated whose need for information provided much of the inspiration for this book. Finally, we would like to express our thanks to our colleagues on the staff and faculty at the United States Military Academy for their unwavering commitment to the pursuit of knowledge. Seldom does one have the opportunity to work in an environment and with colleagues who by their presence serve as a continuing source of motivation and inspiration.

INTRODUCTION

"Your lot is mortal: not mortal is what you desire."

— Ovid

Each of us became deeply involved with the treatment and prevention of back pain in a different way. One became involved as a natural outgrowth of his professional responsibilities as an orthopedic surgeon assigned to Keller Army Hospital at the United States Military Academy at West Point, New York, where he annually sees hundreds of patients suffering from back pain. The other became interested nearly eight years ago when he first suffered a bout of back pain. Quite frankly, before his unwelcomed initiation into the world of back pain, he had never given the matter much thought. In retrospect, given his profession and his responsibilities for the physical training of the Corps of Cadets, his failure to acknowledge back pain as a serious problem that affects members of our society in all walks of life was a regrettable oversight.

With our diverse backgrounds and perspectives, some may wonder how we got together to share ideas on treating back pain and why we undertook the collaborative effort that resulted in this book. The answer to both questions is relatively simple: We share a mutual concern for the health and welfare of the members of the West Point community—the cadets, staff and faculty, support personnel and dependents. Despite the strong community-wide emphasis on fitness and wellness, West Point has a pattern of serious back pain suffering similar to that in most communities. Even among the Corps of Cadets—probably the most physically fit college-age student body anywhere—the incidence of back pain is great. Moreover, the intense physical demands of a career as an officer in the United States Army make such a condition even more intolerable. As a result, we both have spent considerable effort and energy in an attempt to better understand the causes of back pain so that we might identify more effective and efficient methods for dealing with it.

As you will read in this book, medicine is not an exact science. Understandably, this is not the best news for those who suffer from back pain. If members of the medical community cannot agree on what is wrong with back pain sufferers and how to treat them, is it any wonder that literally millions of back pain sufferers face what they perceive to be a hopeless situation?

This book was developed in an attempt to at least partially rectify that dilemma. Actually, *The Goodbye Back Pain Handbook* was written to serve three objectives. *First,* we want to provide an overview of the basic information you should know about your back. Certainly, more technical and more comprehensive explanations of how the back works and why it may not work properly have been penned. At some point, however, the information can become so complex and so overbearing as to divert your willingness or ability to adequately comprehend what you are reading. For those who would like a thorough description of the anatomy of the back, the bibliography at the end of the book provides suggestions for additional reading material. *Second,* for the first time in print, the BackMate® protocol for treating back pain is explained. The BackMate was developed at West Point and successfully tested on over 200 members of the West Point community, as well as in two formal research studies, one with executives at the Pepsi Cola Worldwide Headquarters and one at the New York School of Medicine. The revolutionary BackMate protocol has been found to be the most effective method ever discovered for stretching and strengthening the musculature of the lower back. *Third,* the book attempts to crack the veneer of hopelessness facing many back pain sufferers. Your back pain can and should be treated. This book is an essential first step in that treatment.

Chapter 1 presents an overview of the anatomy of the back. Chapter 2 offers a synopsis of the most common causes of back pain. An explanation of how back pain is diagnosed and evaluated is included in Chapter 3. Chapter 4 discusses how each person can treat his back pain. The BackMate protocol is described in Chapter 5. Chapter 6 offers common-sense suggestions on how best to prevent back pain from occurring. Finally, Chapter 7 includes some of the most commonly asked questions regarding back pain and the answers to each inquiry.

It is certainly a natural inclination, before reading further, to ask yourself the following question: "Will reading this book and following the advice included in it guarantee that my back will get better?" In all honesty, no one – including the two of us – can make that guarantee. What we've presented in this book is our best opinion, based upon the most current information available and our years of firsthand experience with those who suffer from back pain. While we feel strongly that the information in this book is the best advice we can offer, ultimately you must assume full responsibility for whatever course of action you decide to take. If our advice differs from that of your doctor, we suggest that you either follow the suggestions of your own physician, who obviously has the advantage of having examined you and knowing your unique situation, or consult another doctor for another opinion.

Other than accentuating your feelings of relief when you're not experiencing it, back pain has absolutely no redeeming value. *The Goodbye Back Pain Handbook* was written to enable you to say, "Goodbye back pain, hello life." Simply reading this book, however, won't make your back pain go away. Despite the mild disclaimer in the previous paragraph, we strongly recommend that you follow the suggestions we offer in this book. Keep in mind that if you sincerely want your back pain to "go away," it is absolutely critical that you closely adhere to proper back care techniques. Mix in a reasonable measure of common sense and a dash of plain old hard work, and you've got a great chance to succeed. We wish you luck.

James A. Peterson, Ph.D.

James Wheeler, M.D.

The
GOODBYE
BACK PAIN
Handbook

1

YOUR BACK: AN ANATOMICAL OVERVIEW

"If anything is sacred, the human body is sacred."

– Walt Whitman

When someone is called the "backbone" of an organization, it is obvious that that individual is vital to the health and well-being of that organization. Similarly, the human backbone is vital to the health and well-being of each person. Your backbone is the basic *support* system that connects your upper body with your lower body, allowing you to sit, stand upright, work, walk, run and jump. It also serves the important function of *protection* for your spinal cord. In addition to support and protection, the backbone is flexible so that *motion* can occur. Providing support, protection and the flexibility for motion, your backbone easily qualifies as one of the most vital components of your good health and well-being (Figure 1–1).

When this vital component is not working and causes you pain and distress, you obviously want to know why, and you want to know what you can do to remedy the situation. However, before you can understand why your back doesn't work properly, you must understand how it is supposed to function, and that requires some knowledge of the anatomy of the spine. Your spine is made of many parts, all working together. A problem with any one of the individual parts can lead to dysfunction of your entire spine.

3

SUPPORT   PROTECTION   MOTION

Figure 1–1   Functions of the backbone

The spine has three basic components: 1) the bony framework (bones, ligaments and discs), 2) the spinal cord (and nerves) and 3) the muscles. By becoming familiar with the anatomy of the basic parts of your spine, you will be better able to understand how each component functions individually and how all the components function together.

THE BONY FRAMEWORK: BONES, DISCS AND LIGAMENTS

Bones

Your backbone is made up of 24 individual bones located between your skull and your pelvis, plus the sacrum and the coccyx (Figure 1–2). These bones are called vertebrae and are connected by discs and ligaments. The vertebrae are named according to their location in the spine. The upper seven vertebrae are known as the cervical vertebrae of the neck (C1 – C7), and the lower five vertebrae are called the lumbar vertebrae of the lower back (L1 – L5).   In between are the 12 thoracic vertebrae, to which the ribs are attached (T1 – T12).

The last lumbar vertebrae (L5) sits on top of your sacrum. The sacrum is a broad, triangular, bony structure composed of five vertebrae that fused together into a single bone during the first few months of your life. The sacrum is designed to provide rigid support for your pelvis. Your coccyx is a collection of three or four small vertebrae fused into a single vertebra. It is frequently referred to as the "tailbone," since it is probably the remnant of what once was mankind's tail. About two inches long, your coccyx attaches to the lower point of your sacrum. It provides an anchorage for several of the small muscles in your rectal area that are essential to the control of bowel movement.

When viewed from behind, your spine should be straight (Figure 1–2). When viewed from the side, the vertebrae are aligned so that your spine has a gentle lazy S curve to it. This curve is formed by a forward bend of your spine in the cervical and lumbar areas and a backward bend in the thoracic area. These curves balance each other so that your head is centered over your pelvis.

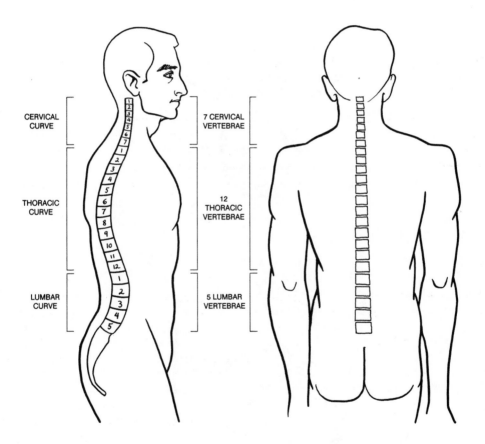

Figure 1–2   The backbone: side and back views

The vertebrae form a protective ring around the spinal cord. The center of this ring is called the spinal canal because it is the canal through which your spinal cord passes. The anatomy of this protective ring can be best appreciated by looking at an individual vertebra from above (Figure 1–3). The ring of bone is formed by the vertebral body in front, the pedicles on the side and the lamina in back. Each vertebra also has a spinous process and two transverse processes to which ligaments, muscles and ribs attach. Looking at a vertebra from the side, you can see that each vertebra is connected to the vertebra above and below it by its facet joints and by a disc. The opening on the side of each vertebra is for the spinal nerves to exit the protective bony framework of the spine.

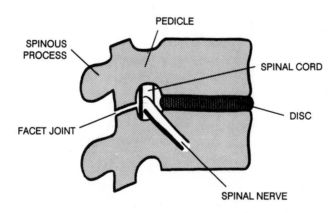

Figure 1–3 Vertebra: from above (top) and from the side (bottom).

Discs

Discs are structures between adjoining vertebrae. "Disc" is an appropriate descriptive term because each disc has a flat, circular shape (Figure 1–4). Discs are made of a cartilage material similar in consistency to rubber, and they function as the shock absorbers of the spine.

Each disc has a semisolid center (nucleus) that is supported by a ring of tissue (annulus) that surrounds this center. The center of the disc is mainly responsible for the shock absorbing properties of the disc, and the ring of tissue is the support that prevents the disc from collapsing.

Figure 1–4   Two side views of discs, illustrating their shock-absorbing properties, and a disc viewed from above

Ligaments

Ligaments are strong bands of fibrous connective tissue that function to hold bones together. Each joint in your body is formed by two bones held together by ligaments.

Whereas ligaments are strong enough to hold joints together, they are also flexible and elastic enough to allow controlled motion in a joint. If a ligament is torn, however, excessive motion can occur, and a joint can be dislocated.

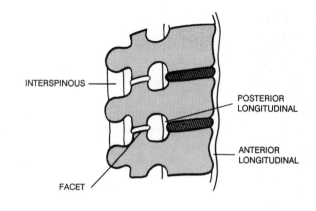

In the spine, the ligaments function to hold the vertebrae together, and there are several ligaments in your spine that connect each vertebra to the one above and below it (Figure 1-5). The only direct

Figure 1-5 Ligaments of the spine

bone-to-bone connection between adjoining vertebrae is the facet joints, which are held together by ligaments. Although there is some motion between the vertebral bodies where they come into contact with the discs, it is at the facet joints where the majority of spinal motion occurs. The connection of the vertebral bodies to each other through the disc is supported by the anterior and posterior longitudinal ligaments. These ligaments extend from the top of your spine down to your sacrum, with one at the front and the other at the back of the vertebral body. The posterior ligament separates the bodies of the vertebrae from your spinal canal. Additional stability is provided by the interspinous ligaments, which extend from the spinous process of one vertebrae to the spinous process of the next, down the entire length of your spine, and by the ligamentum flavum, which connects lamina to lamina.

THE SPINAL CORD

Your spinal cord is a direct extension of your brain and is responsible for carrying messages from your brain to your body and from your body back to your brain (Figure 1-6). These messages are transmitted through nerves in a fashion similar to the conduction of electricity through telephone wires. A nerve has two basic functions: motor and sensory. The motor nerves are responsible for activating muscle groups or organs to perform certain actions. The sensory nerves provide input to your brain from your body. The combination of sensory input and motor output allows your body (using its brain, spinal cord and nerves) to respond appropriately to external stimuli.

To illustrate sensory and motor interactions, consider the following example. If you touch a hot stove with your hand, a sensory nerve takes that information to your spinal cord, which transmits it to your brain. Your brain then interprets that information and sends a message down through your spinal cord to a motor nerve, which activates the muscle group that pulls your hand away from the stove. You can appreciate how fast this sensory input and motor output process occurs when you consider how quickly you pull your hand away from the stove.

The human nervous system (brain, spinal cord and nerves) is magnificent in the way it works, but it is also very fragile and needs very good protection. The skull is made of hard bone to protect your brain, and the backbone protects your spinal cord.

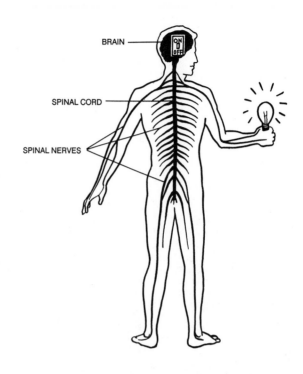

Figure 1–6 The brain, spinal cord and nerves

THE SPINAL MUSCLES

The 140 muscles that run along the back of your spine from the base of your skull to your pelvis and attach to your spine are called the spinal muscles. These muscles perform a substantial amount of work. Other muscles aid the spinal muscles in supporting your spine. The abdominal muscles are very important in supporting your spine, much more so than most people realize. They are so important that they could be considered the "anterior spinal muscles." The muscles of your pelvis, hips and upper legs, including the buttock, hamstring and quadriceps muscles also directly or indirectly support your spine.

The framework of your spine is provided by the vertebral bones held together by ligaments and discs, but it is your muscles that support that framework and provide the means for motion (Figure 1–7). If, for example, you become paralyzed, even though your bones and ligaments are functional, you will be unable to stand erect because your do not have functioning muscles. Similarly, when you faint, you will fall to the ground because all your muscles have stopped working momentarily. Muscles and the voluntary control that you have over them give you the ability to stand erect and move about.

Figure 1–7   The spinal muscles: side view (left), back view (right)

FUNCTION

As stated before, your spine is a well-constructed system that connects and *supports* your upper and your lower body, provides *protection* for your spinal cord, but yet allows flexibility and *motion.* For these functions of support, protection and motion to be effectively and painlessly accomplished, all the components of your spine must be in good working order.

The bones in your back are the foundation or building blocks of your spine, held together by ligaments and discs, with motion occurring from the action of your muscles. A healthy back is sturdy and strong for support and protection, but it is also flexible so that motion can occur.

THE NEXT STEP

The preceding section on the anatomy of your back was designed to provide you with an abbreviated overview of how your back works. Chapter 2 examines the causes of back pain. We recommend that, when necessary, you refer back to this chapter for an explanation of the basic back anatomy. The effort will be worthwhile. Comprehending what is wrong with your back and what to do about it will be easier if you understand how your back functions normally.

2

THE CAUSES OF BACK PAIN

"Your cause is hidden but the result is well known."

– Ovid

Humans are more prone to back pain than four-legged animals, because they stand in an upright position and transmit the gravitational forces on their spines to two legs rather than four legs. This increase of the natural forces of gravity is concentrated in the lower spine area. Somewhat understandably, it is the lower spine that is the source of most back pain.

To understand what causes back pain, you must have an insight into the spine's anatomy. Briefly, your vertebral bones are the framework of the spine that protects your spinal cord and the nerves coming from it. Your vertebrae are held together by ligaments and discs, and the motion of the vertebrae is controlled by muscles. Problems with any one of these structures (vertebrae, ligaments, discs, muscles, spinal cord or nerves) can cause back pain. This chapter examines the common and the not-so-common causes of back pain and attempts to explain why some people have back pain with no apparent cause.

CATEGORIZING BACK PAIN

Back pain has traditionally been described and categorized in a number of ways. We recommend categorizing back pain on the basis of two broad parameters. The system we advocate is based on an attempt to simplify the description and categorization process for back pain in terms that most individuals can understand.

First, we describe back pain by the length of time it has been present. Back pain that started recently (days, to a few weeks ago) is termed *acute,* and back pain of a repetitive, long-standing nature is called *chronic.*

Second, we further describe back pain by the basic mechanism causing the pain without referring to any specific anatomical structure. There are two basic mechanisms of back pain: traumatic and degenerative. *Traumatic* infers that some injury or injuries are the basic cause of the pain, whereas *degenerative* indicates that arthritis or the normal aging process is the primary cause of the back pain. Although there are many *other,* less common causes of back pain (some of which will be discussed later in this chapter), the two most common mechanisms are traumatic and degenerative.

Explaining back pain when there is no mechanism or cause is not as easy. We use the term *idiopathic* to define back pain that apparently normal people have when there is no obvious reason for the pain and when the other causes of back pain have been excluded.

Back pain, then, can be grouped into four basic categories: 1) traumatic, 2) degenerative, 3) idiopathic and 4) other. Table 2–1 is a listing of the basic categories of back pain and includes examples of the basic causes of back pain associated with each category. Traumatic, degenerative and idiopathic back pain are discussed in some detail in subsequent sections, followed by an abbreviated overview of several of the causes designated as *other* back pain.

---

1. **TRAUMATIC BACK PAIN**
   - Fractured bones
   - Sprained ligaments
   - Strained muscles
   - Disc injuries

2. **DEGENERATIVE BACK PAIN**
   - Degenerative arthritis
   - Degenerative discs
   - Spinal stenosis

3. **IDIOPATHIC BACK PAIN**
   - "Everday" back pain in healthy people
   - Poor posture — excess weight
   - Pregnancy
   - Overuse injuries
   - Poor flexibility — hamstring tightness

4. **OTHER CAUSES OF BACK PAIN**
   - Developmental (scoliosis, kyphosis, lordosis, spondylolisthesis)
   - Inflammatory (rheumatoid arthritis, ankylosing, spondylitis)
   - Infection
   - Neoplastic (tumors)
   - Metabolic (osteoporosis)

Table 2–1 Causes of back pain

TRAUMATIC BACK PAIN

Everyone can relate to *fractured* wrist bones, *sprained* ankle ligaments and a *strained* leg muscle. These types of injuries can also occur in the bones, ligaments and muscles of your back, either singly or in combination with one another. Unfortunately, we are not as familiar with our back as we are with our arms and legs (we need a mirror just to see our back). For this reason, we sometimes have difficulty understanding that a sprained or injured back can be caused by the same things that cause a sprained or injured leg muscle. In addition, traumatic back pain can be caused by *discs* that *rupture* or *herniate*.

Any injury can be *acute*, which means that the injury recently occurred. On the other hand, an injury can be *chronic* in nature, meaning that over the months or years, several or many injuries have occurred. A chronic injury may be a significant injury but, more commonly, it is an accumulation of milder injuries.

Fractured Bones

Just as you can fall and fracture bones in your wrist, you can also fracture the bones of your spine (vertebrae). Thankfully, however, fractures of the vertebrae are not nearly as common as fractures of other bones in your body. In fact, fractures of the spinal bones are unusual in healthy people, and they occur most often as a result of a significant injury, such as a bad fall or a car accident.

Your spine is a very well-constructed support system that can absorb a great deal of shock or impact without fracturing the bones because the discs between the vertebrae protect the bones of the spine. You can imagine how fragile we would be without these built-in shock absorbers. Injuries to the discs are far more common than fractures of the spine. This is important to know, because a fracture of your spine that causes a displacement or shattering of the bones could lead to an injury to your spinal cord and possible paralysis.

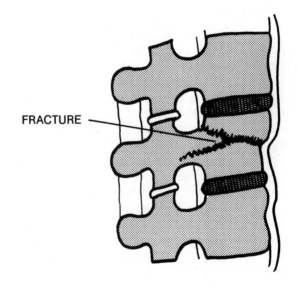

FRACTURE

Figure 2–1 A fractured bone

Sprained Ligaments and Strained Muscles

The most common injuries of the spine are not injuries to the bones or discs but rather injuries to the ligaments (sprains) and muscles (strains). The mechanisms of sprained ligaments and strained muscles in the spine are similar to the mechanisms of injuries that occur elsewhere in your body. For example, athletes can strain a leg muscle running, or they can strain a back muscle while lifting too much. Basketball players can twist and sprain their ankles, or they can twist and sprain their backs. Because the ligaments and muscles of your spine are so close to each other, however, it may not be as easy to differentiate between injuries to the ligaments and injuries to the muscles of your back as it is elsewhere in your body.

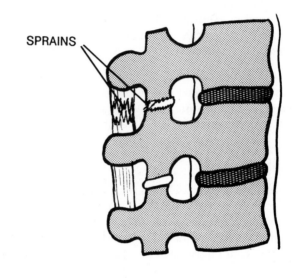

Figure 2–2 Sprained ligaments

A sprained ligament occurs when it is stretched beyond its normal fixed length, such as can happen with sudden or violent bending or twisting. When you use your back to lift or move, motion occurs between each vertebra. The ligaments function as check-reins or tie-downs to prevent excessive motion. When the maximum allowable motion has occurred, the ligament becomes taut. The ligaments have some elasticity and the ability to stretch a small amount, but not a great deal. A sprained ligament can vary from very mild to severe. A sprain is classified as mild when there is no significant damage to the ligament. In a mild sprain, pain occurs when that ligament is stretched, although the pain may not be present until the day after the injury. A severe sprain means that the ligament has been damaged or torn. In this instance the pain will be much worse and recovery longer. When an injury occurs to a ligament in your spine, any motion of that injured area will stress the injured ligament and be very painful. As a result, your sprained back becomes stiff and painful to move.

If a ligament has been torn, it will heal, but it may not be as taut as it was originally. Part of the healing process includes the formation of scar tissue, which is not as strong as normal ligamentous tissue and is less flexible. A healed torn ligament therefore is not as tight, not as strong and not as flexible as an uninjured ligament. As a result, that ligament is more likely to be reinjured and probably will be.

A strained muscle ("pulled muscle," "charley horse") most often occurs when a muscle is stressed beyond its capability to contract, such as when a back muscle is strained when you lift something too heavy or lift something in an improper manner. A muscle strain can also occur when a relaxed or partially relaxed muscle is suddenly or unexpectedly overstretched. Whereas ligaments have a relatively fixed length, the length of a muscle changes markedly depending on the degree of contraction. The ability to voluntarily contract or relax skeletal muscles gives you the ability to control the motion in your joints.

Muscle strains vary from mild to severe depending on the amount of damage to the muscle unit. In a mild strain, there is no appreciable damage to the muscle, and, although the muscle is able to function, you experience pain when you use it. The pain may not occur until the day following the injury after the muscle has tightened or stiffened up. In a severe strain, there is a tear of the muscle that is accompanied by significant pain and dysfunction.

A muscle spasm may occur after a muscle has been injured. A muscle tightens up, or goes into spasm, as a way of protecting itself from further overstretching and further injury. Muscle spasm can also occur after another structure near the muscle (a ligament, bone or disc) has been injured. This muscle spasm occurs because the muscles become secondarily irritated by the injury or because the muscles are trying to protect the injured area. When a muscle goes into spasm, motion around that injured area is decreased, protecting that area from further injury and from motion that would be painful.

As a muscle strain heals, the pain and spasm associated with it will subside. If there has been a tear in the muscle, the healing process includes formation of some scar tissue in the injured area. The scar tissue formed is not as elastic as normal muscle tissue, and the muscle may lose some of its ability to relax and contract. This loss of elasticity makes that muscle more prone to future injury.

Proper conditioning and stretching out before and after physical activity make muscles less prone to injury. Most competitive athletes are aware not only of the benefits, but also of the necessities of proper training and stretching techniques in preventing muscle strains. Once a muscle has been injured, conditioning and stretching are even more important in preventing future injuries.

Disc Injuries

Many terms are used in discussing disc injuries, including "slipped," "bulging," "ruptured" and "herniated." You should not be confused by these different terms, as each term is a fairly accurate description of what has actually happened to the disc.

A slipped or bulging disc is a disc that has slipped out or is bulging from between the vertebrae (Figure 2–3). A ruptured disc is a disc in which the supporting ring of tissue around the center of the disc has been disrupted. If the injury is carried one step further, the disc material in the center of the disc can herniate through the rupture in the supporting ring of tissue (Figure 2–4).

Figure 2–3   Disc injuries

NORMAL DISC
— NUCLEUS
— ANNULUS

BULGING DISC

RUPTURED DISC

HERNIATED DISC

Figure 2–4   A herniated disc

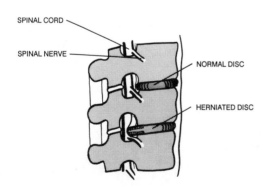

SPINAL CORD

SPINAL NERVE

NORMAL DISC

HERNIATED DISC

An injury to the disc itself (and the ligaments supporting it) can be a source of pain. If the disc has ruptured and disc material has herniated, pain can come not only from the area of the injured disc, but also from the disc material pressing on the spinal cord and the surrounding nerves. The nerve most commonly affected in disc injuries is the sciatic nerve. When a herniated disc puts pressure on the sciatic nerve, the nerve becomes irritated and sciatica results. Sciatica is a sharp, intense and often electric-type shooting pain that starts in your back and travels along the course of the sciatic nerve through your buttocks and the back of your leg to your foot.

DEGENERATIVE BACK PAIN

Unfortunately, the spine, especially the lower spine, goes through a normal aging or degeneration process that is probably accelerated in animals walking on two, rather than four, legs. Just as "old age" arthritis sets in in our knees or hips, it can also affect the bones of the spine. In fact, if several elderly individuals were to have an X-ray made of the lumbar region of the spine, most, if not all, would have at least some degenerative arthritic changes present on that X-ray. This doesn't mean, however, that all of these individuals have back pain. What it does mean is that the degenerative process involving the bones and discs is part of the normal aging process.

Degenerative Arthritis

Degenerative arthritis of the vertebral bones is similar to the "wear and tear" arthritis that occurs in other joints of your body. With this wear and tear comes inflammation, to which your body may respond by producing bone spurs. This inflammation and bone spur formation can be a source of pain in themselves or can cause pain by irritating other structures of your spine, such as the ligaments, muscles, spinal cord or surrounding nerves.

Degenerative arthritis in the spine occurs in the joints of the spine, primarily in the facet joints and between the vertebral bodies. The pain of degenerative arthritis in your spine is similar to arthritic pain in other joints of your body. This pain is occasionally sharp, but more often it is dull and aching. Arthritic pain is aggravated by cold weather or weather changes. Since arthritic pain is also aggravated by inactivity, it is common to experience pain and stiffness in the mornings.

Figure 2–5 Characteristic stance of a person with degenerative arthritis

Degenerative Discs

Degenerative discs and degenerative arthritis of the spine usually accompany each other. The degenerative aging process that affects the vertebrae also affects their shock absorbers, the discs. The discs are made of a cartilage substance similar in

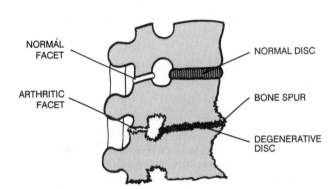

Figure 2–6   Causes of degenerative back pain: degenerative arthritis and degenerative discs

NORMAL FACET

ARTHRITIC FACET

NORMAL DISC

BONE SPUR

DEGENERATIVE DISC

consistency to hard rubber. With increasing age, the water content of these discs decreases and, as a result, the discs flatten and lose their shock absorbing capacity (Figure 2–6). A disc degenerates slowly over a period of time. A degenerative disc usually is referred to as a flattened or bulging disc, not as a ruptured or herniated disc that is traumatic in origin.

The pain of a degenerative disc is similar to the dull, aching pain of degenerative arthritis. A degenerative disc can put pressure on your spinal cord and nerves. Because the formation of a degenerative disc is such a gradual process, however, you may not remember when you initially experienced the pain. The leg pain of a degenerative disc is not as sharp or well-defined as the pain of sciatica (the sharp pain felt down your leg) from a herniated disc. Those with a herniated disc can usually remember the day their sciatic pain started, but those with a degenerative disc will speak in months or years when asked when their back or leg pain started.

Spinal Stenosis

Spinal stenosis is the term that is used to describe the narrowing of the spinal canal (carrying the spinal cord and nerves). Any condition that narrows the spinal canal (a herniated disc, for example) is, in effect, spinal stenosis (Figure 2–7). The term spinal stenosis, however, usually refers to the narrowing of the spinal canal that is associated with degenerative arthritis and degenerative discs.

Spinal stenosis is a degenerative process associated with aging. Not surprisingly, most patients with spinal stenosis are over age 50. The arthritis that is present in the facet joints and between the vertebral bodies causes bone spur formation. This arthritis, along with degenerative bulging discs, combines to narrow the cross sectional area of the spinal canal and put pressure on the spinal cord and nerves.

A combination of back and leg pain is the result of spinal stenosis. The back pain is similar to the chronic, aching pain of degenerative arthritis. The leg pain is similar to the leg pain associated with degenerative discs and is caused by pressure on the spinal cord and nerves. The leg pain of spinal stenosis may be quite vague. It is sometimes blamed on poor circulation because it comes on after physical activity. If you experience spinal stenosis, you soon learn how far you can walk before your legs start hurting and how long they take to stop hurting when you rest.

Spinal stenosis is suspected when someone over the age of 50 has a somewhat vague history of back and leg pain, doesn't have any dramatic physical findings on examination, but does have arthritis on regular X–rays. The diagnosis is confirmed by CAT scan and myelography.

Figure 2–7 Spinal stenosis

IDIOPATHIC BACK PAIN
("EVERYDAY" BACK PAIN IN HEALTHY PEOPLE)

It is easy to understand why someone has back pain after they have had an injury to their back. It is also relatively easy to explain to elderly individuals that their back pain is caused by arthritis in their spine. It is not so easy, however, to explain why healthy, young individuals have back pain when they are physically fit and have never had a back injury.

Unfortunately, it is "normal" for healthy, young people to have back pain at some point, and, in fact, almost everyone has experienced or will experience back pain during their lifetime. About one-half of the working force is unable to go to work because of back pain at some time in their lives.

The previous sections discussed traumatic and degenerative back pain. The third, and perhaps most common, grouping of back pain is idiopathic. This category concerns back pain in otherwise fit and healthy people.

Idiopathic is a word that means "no known cause." The term "idiopathic back pain" is used to categorize that group of people who have back pain, but don't have a good reason for it and don't fall into one of the other three categories of back pain (traumatic, degenerative or other). There are several factors in idiopathic back pain that may predispose an otherwise healthy person to back pain. These include the effects of poor posture and excess weight, pregnancy, overuse injuries and poor flexibility and tight hamstring muscles.

Poor Posture and Excess Weight

Poor posture or excess weight in themselves will not cause back pain overnight, nor will they necessarily ever cause back pain. Long-standing poor posture and excess weight, however, increase the forces on your spine and can accelerate the degenerative changes that are inevitable with age. As mentioned previously, humans walking on two legs in an upright position already have more forces placed on their spine than do four-legged animals.

The human spine when viewed from the side curves in a gentle, lazy S shape. Poor posture and excess weight increase the curves that are normally present, causing kyphosis (an increase in the thoracic curve) and lordosis (an increase in the lumbar curve). Changing the spinal curves increases the forces and stresses on your vertebrae, discs, ligaments and muscles (Figure 2–8).

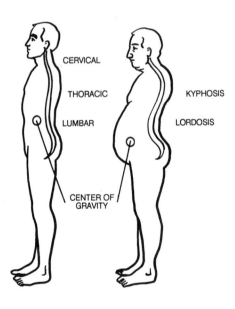

Figure 2–8 The effects of poor posture and excess weight

NORMAL CURVES   ABNORMAL CURVES

Prolonged bad posture and excess weight also place all of the components of your spine at risk for injury and pain. Because your vertebrae and discs have increased forces put on them, they are more susceptible to degenerative changes. Your ligaments also incur increased stresses. As a result, they are more prone to chronic injury. Your muscles are put at a mechanical disadvantage, forcing them to work harder to accomplish the same amount of work or causing them to become lazy in the position of poor posture. Either way, they are more prone to chronic injury.

Those who don't think that excess weight or a big, protruding belly can aggravate or cause back pain should fill their pockets with lead, strap a bowling ball to their belly and wear a backpack every day for several years. Not only will their back likely hurt, but so will their hips, knees and ankles.

Pregnancy

Pregnancy is an example of an increase in abdominal weight that causes a change in posture, increases forces on the spine and predisposes the pregnant female to back pain. Placing the pregnant female in the same category as the overweight poor-postured individual is not quite fair, however, but as far as the spine is concerned, the same basic process occurs.

The excess lower abdominal weight, especially later in the pregnancy, has a similar effect on the spine as excess weight and poor posture in nonpregnant people. The additional weight causes an increase in the curve normally present in the lumbar spine (lordosis). The change in this curve and the additional body weight places increased forces and stresses on the vertebrae, discs, ligaments and muscles of the spine. As a result, the components of the spine are more susceptible to fatigue, injury and pain.

Back pain does not necessarily accompany pregnancy, but pregnancy does place the back at an increased risk for pain. If you experienced back pain before and become pregnant, the chances are even greater that you will have more back pain during your pregnancy.

Overuse Injuries

Overuse injuries in athletes, especially runners, are a well-known problem. Because we are not as familiar with the anatomy or function of our back as we are of our extremities, it is not as well-understood or accepted why we can get overuse problems with our back.

All parts of our body, including our back, have a certain limit of activity that they can endure before problems arise. Different people have different limits, but everyone eventually reaches the point of overuse. Conditioned marathon runners may not reach this limit until they are running 25 miles every day, whereas individuals just starting a running program may encounter problems after running their first mile. Most of you can remember your healthy years as a child when you could play outside all day long every day. Now, as a weekend athlete, you often go to work on Mondays painfully sore from the activities of your weekend.

If weekend athletes have back pain on Mondays, it is usually because they have overused the muscles and other spinal components on the weekend that they had underused the rest of the week. Overuse and underuse are terms relative to whatever "normal" use is. As a "normally active" person, you are susceptible to overuse injuries from athletics. You are also susceptible to overuse injuries in your back from the activities of daily life, including sitting, standing, walking, bending and lifting. A common overuse back pain is the pain that the secretary-typist gets from sitting at her desk all day long. Sitting with an erect, rigid spine stresses the muscles and other components of the spine, eventually causing fatigue, stiffness and pain.

Listing possible overuse problems of the spine is an endless task. Everyone – the weekend athlete, the everyday athlete, the white collar or blue collar worker – is a potential victim of back pain from overuse or underuse. A strong and healthy back needs to be used to remain strong and healthy. You should remember, however, that there is a fine line between using your back, overusing it and underusing it.

Poor Flexibility and Hamstring Tightness

For any muscle or joint to be healthy and functioning, it needs to be strong and flexible. This applies to your back, the muscles of your back and the muscles that directly or indirectly support your back – especially your hamstring muscles. A vicious cycle can begin and perpetuate itself when a normal muscle or joint is just a little stiff and sore from being used or has a minor injury. In order to protect this muscle or joint, you don't use it through its normal range of motion. When you eventually do try to use it, it is still sore because it is still stiff. As time goes on, it becomes more stiff (loses flexibility), becomes more difficult to function normally and becomes more prone to injury, which causes more loss of flexibility, more loss of function and so on. As you can see, a vicious cycle is set in motion.

Flexibility plays an important part in recovering from back pain and in preventing back pain from recurring. Following an episode of back pain, no matter what the cause, you must regain the flexibility in your back and hamstring muscles so that your back can function normally. If you do not restore your level of flexibility, your back will not function normally and will be more prone to future problems, including the recurrence of back pain.

There are some of us who are normally very flexible ("double jointed"), just as there are some of us who are not very flexible. The young gymnast can bend over and touch her palms to the floor without difficulty, but the husky young weightlifter may be able to bend over and only touch his fingertips to his knees. Does an inherent lack of flexibility make someone more prone to back pain? And, if someone has back pain and a lack of flexibility, which condition came first? Did the lack of flexibility cause the back pain, or did the pain cause the lack of flexibility? Regardless of which came first, lack of flexibility or back pain, it is obvious that they are closely related because often when one disappears, so will the other.

A common problem in people with low back pain is tightness of the hamstring muscles, the powerful muscles in the back of the thigh. A measure commonly used to evaluate back pain is the straight leg test (discussed further in Chapter 3). In this test you lie flat on your back with your legs straight. The doctor then lifts one of your legs off the table and raises it as far as possible. Normally, your leg should be able to be raised to an angle of 90 degrees from the horizontal. Problems that cause a limit in the straight leg test include back pain, disc problems and tight hamstrings. This test demonstrates the interrelationship between back pain and tight hamstrings.

Lack of flexibility in your hamstring muscles can by itself be a significant contributing factor to back pain, or it can be secondary to the pain in your back. Either way, maintaining or gaining flexibility in your hamstring muscles is an important part of the prevention or treatment of back pain. An especially effective means of gaining and maintaining hamstring flexibility is the BackMate apparatus (refer to Chapter 5 for a comprehensive discussion of the use and benefits of BackMate).

OTHER CAUSES OF BACK PAIN

Although the main causes of back pain are traumatic, degenerative or idiopathic in origin, a number of other factors or conditions may also cause back pain. For simplicity's sake, we have grouped them under the title "other causes." These other causes occur less frequently than traumatic, degenerative or idiopathic back pain and are significantly different in origin. Included in this category are developmental back pain, inflammatory back pain, back pain from infection, back pain from neoplasm (tumor) and metabolic back pain.

Developmental Back Pain

The fetal development of the spine and its components is quite complex. Congenital abnormalities of the spine vary from insignificant problems to major defects in the spinal bones or spinal cord and nerves. Abnormalities that develop with growth can likewise vary from mild to severe. They may be associated with no pain, or they may be the cause of disabling back pain.

As the spine grows and develops, especially during the growth spurts of childhood and adolescence, problems can occur. As mentioned, the spine viewed from behind is straight and when viewed from the side has a lazy S curve to it. When viewing the spine from the side, *kyphosis* or round back is an increased angulation in the mid-thoracic spine, whereas *lordosis* is an increased angulation of the lower spine (Figure 2–8). *Scoliosis* is a lateral or "sideways" curvature of the spine as seen when it is viewed from behind (Figure 2–9). These conditions may have no discernible cause (idiopathic), or there may be a localized or generalized growth abnormality.

Figure 2–9 Scoliosis (curvature of the spine)

An example of a localized developmental abnormality is *spondylolysis,* which is a defect in the bony architecture of the spine that may allow forward slipping (*spondylolisthesis*) of one vertebrae on another (Figure 2–10). This condition can lead to hyperlordosis and, if it is severe enough, it can result in pinching of the spinal cord and nerves. Spondylolisthesis can be caused by a fracture in the spine, but more often it is an unrecognized, not completely understood, developmental process that occurs in the growing child.

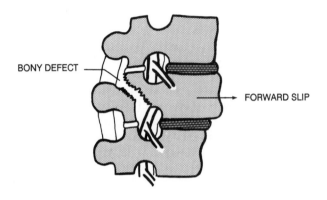

Figure 2–10 Spondylolysis and spondylolisthesis

Inflammatory Back Pain

The word arthritis means inflammation of a joint. Osteoarthritis refers to the degenerative arthritis that occurs as part of the normal aging process or following an injury. Inflammatory arthritis refers to those conditions such as *rheumatoid arthritis* and *ankylosing spondylitis* that can affect the joints of the body, including the spine (Figure 2–11).

Inflammation occurs in all arthritis. In osteoarthritis, the inflammation is secondary to the degenerative process. In inflammatory arthritis, the inflammation itself is the primary process and the cause of pain or dysfunction.

The back pain of inflammatory arthritis is often similar to degenerative back pain in that it comes on slowly and progressively, but there is no history of a significant injury. In addition, inflammatory arthritis usually occurs at an earlier age and is often associated with inflammatory joint problems. Conditions such as rheumatoid arthritis and ankylosing spondylitis can be detected with blood tests.

Figure 2-11 Inflammatory back pain: rheumatoid arthritis (left) and ankylosing spondylitis (right)

Back Pain from Infection

Infection is a rare cause of back pain and can involve the vertebrae, the discs or the spinal cord (meningitis). Infection can spread from other parts of the body through the bloodstream to the spine. In children, spinal infections usually follow respiratory tract infections. In adults, spinal infections may follow kidney or urinary tract infections. Infections can also occur after spinal surgery.

Back Pain from Neoplasm (Tumor)

Abnormal tumors or growths—cancerous or noncancerous—can involve your spine and any of its components and cause back pain. These growths can originate in your spine or spread to your spine from a cancerous tumor elsewhere in your body.

Metabolic Back Pain

Metabolic causes of back pain are those that result in abnormal or insufficient bone. A common metabolic cause of back pain is *osteoporosis.* Osteoporosis is a decrease in the mineral substance of bone that results in a weakening of the bone. It occurs most commonly in elderly people, especially post-menopausal women. This process, to a certain extent, normally occurs later in life, but may be accelerated by a combination of hormonal and

Figure 2-12 Metabolic back pain

dietary factors, as well as decreased physical activity. Osteoporosis can be a source of back pain and can also result in vertebral compression fractures. Many other metabolic diseases can cause problems in bone formation, including scurvy, rickets, kidney dysfunction and other hormonal imbalances.

THE NEXT STEP

In our opinion, understanding the cause of your back pain is more important than understanding the specific anatomical structure involved. Once you are aware of the cause of your pain, it is easier to then understand which anatomical structure is involved. The basic causes of back pain were examined in abbreviated detail in this chapter. Keep in mind that the list of potential causes of back pain is almost endless. We've attempted to provide you with an overview of the most common conditions.

In the next chapter, the evaluation process used by physicians to diagnose and evaluate the specific causes of back pain is described, including the typical history and the type of pain usually associated with each cause of back pain.

3

YOU AND YOUR DOCTOR

"Pain is oft a visitant; but pain clings cruelly to us."

–John Keats

If your back pain shows signs of being more that a minor problem, you should see a doctor. For example, if you have persistent pain down one of your arms or legs, it can be more than a minor problem. Your back pain can also be serious if it is accompanied by other symptoms, such as weakness in one of your arms or legs, bowel difficulties or chronic pain. This chapter presents guidelines on selecting a doctor to diagnose and treat your back pain. Also included is an abbreviated overview of the process used by physicians to evaluate your back pain. Finally, suggestions on whether or not you should seek out a second medical opinion on your back pain are presented.

SELECTING A DOCTOR

As a rule, your choice of a physician to treat your back pain will be between a general practice doctor, an orthopedic specialist, a neurosurgeon or neurologist and an osteopath. Many individuals also choose either a physical therapist or a chiropractor to attend to their back pain.

A general practice or family practice doctor is trained to deal with a wide variety of medical problems and patients of all ages. General practitioners are also sources of referrals for patients requiring specialized treatment. Orthopedic specialists are individuals who specialize in bone and joint problems and whose training involves attention to the mechanical, structural and architectural factors relating to your spine. Neurogists and neurosurgeons are specialists in the central and peripheral nervous systems. Osteopaths undergo training generally equivalent to an M.D.'s but with an emphasis on spinal manipulation. Physical therapists are registered health-care technologists who specialize in rehabilitative exercise. Chiropractors are licensed health-care specialists who utilize spinal manipulation as their primary means of therapy.

Not surprisingly, no hard-and-fast rule exists that you can apply to the task of selecting your doctor. Your primary selection criteria must be that the doctor is eminently qualified to make an accurate assessment of your problem and capable of administering the appropriate treatment therapy. The trained specialist you select to treat your back should treat backs on a regular basis and should be thoroughly up to date on the most current information and techniques for treating back pain.

Whereas a physician's reputation and the recommendation of someone whose opinion you respect can guide you to your initial choice of a doctor, you still need to use your own judgment. Knowing as much as possible about how your back works and what the general causes of back pain are can help you proceed more reasonably. A basic understanding of how your doctor will diagnose and evaluate your back pain is invaluable. The more you understand the entire process, including how your back functions and the disorders that impair these functions and cause pain, the better you will be able to decide whether or not your doctor is treating you in a satisfactory manner.

EVALUATING AND DIAGNOSING YOUR BACK PAIN

Having identified the person you would like to serve as your doctor, the next step is to undergo a thorough evaluation. When physicians or health care specialists are evaluating any musculoskeletal problem, be it a knee, ankle, shoulder or back injury, their thought processes are basically the same. First a *history* of the problem is obtained, then a *physical examination* is performed and finally *special studies* such as X-rays are ordered. Each of these three aspects of this investigative effort is important in the overall evaluation of back pain and any other musculoskeletal problem (Figure 3–1). The more thorough the analysis of all aspects of your back problem, the more effective your doctor will be in prescribing proper treatment.

HISTORY

Obtaining a good history from patients about their problems is probably the most important information in the overall investigative process because it is the first step in the evaluation of back pain. Obtaining a history may be simple, or it may require some detective work, but it should at least start off with some very simple information.

Figure 3–1 Evaluating and diagnosing back pain

A history usually involves having the patient complete a written questionnaire. A good history answers the questions: *who, what, where, when, and why.* Table 3–1 presents the histories of three people experiencing back pain:

1. A 16-year-old female gymnast who fell yesterday at practice and now has sharp pain in her low back.

2. A 70-year-old retired accountant who has had dull pain in his low back for 20 years, but can't remember any injury.

3. A 30-year-old healthy recreational athlete who has experienced sharp and dull low back pain off and on for several years but can't recall any injury.

Table 3–1 Three patient histories

WHO? (patient information)	WHAT? (type of pain)	WHERE? (location of pain)	WHEN? (onset of pain)	WHY? (cause of pain)
16-year-old female gymnast	sharp pain	low back	yesterday	injury (traumatic)
70-year-old retired accountant	dull pain	low back	20 years ago	wear and tear (degenerative)
30-year-old healthy recreational athlete	sharp and dull pain	low back	several years ago	??? (idiopathic)

Each of these three people has low back pain, but their stories are significantly different. In each case, a thorough history (answering the simple questions *who, what, where, when* and *why*) makes it easy to see why their stories are different. A good history is the starting point in the evaluation process of their back pain and can even allow us to make some presumptions about the cause of their back pain.

The terms discussed in Chapter 2 that describe the *causes of back pain* are: 1) *traumatic,* 2) *degenerative,* and 3) *idiopathic.* It is easy to categorize each of these three patients into a presumptive category of back pain according to the *cause* of the pain:

1. The 16-year-old gymnast has *traumatic* back pain (Figure 3–2).

2. The 70-year-old retired accountant has *degenerative* back pain (Figure 3–3).

3. The 30-year-old healthy recreational athlete has *idiopathic* back pain (Figure 3–4).

Figure 3–2

Figure 3–3

Figure 3–4

In addition to the cause of the pain, it is important to further investigate the *type* of pain, because this also can be a clue to the origin of the pain. Although it may be difficult to categorize types of pain precisely, *there are three basic types of pain* that occur in your back.

Type 1 pain can be fairly well localized and originates in the superficial structures (skin, spinous processes, interspinal ligaments and spinal muscles). This is the type of pain seen in acute traumatic back pain and is the type of pain that the 16-year-old gymnast is having.

Figure 3–5   Type 1 pain

Type 2 pain is a deep, aching pain, not as well localized as Type 1 pain. It is usually the result of problems in the bony framework of the spine (the vertebrae, facet joints and discs). This pain may radiate into the flanks or buttocks. This is the type of pain seen in chronic traumatic, degenerative or idiopathic back pain and is the type of pain both the 70-year-old accountant and the 30-year-old recreational athlete are having.

Type 3 pain is caused by irritation of the spinal nerves and is intense, sharp and electric in nature. The degree of pain depends on the amount of nerve compression and can cause back pain that shoots into the lower leg or neurologic changes such as a decrease in sensation and strength in the lower leg. This is the type of pain present in sciatica.

Figure 3–6   Type 2 pain

Obviously, these pain patterns overlap and may occur together if there is a combination of problems.

Figure 3–7   Type 3 pain

PHYSICAL EXAMINATION

Just as obtaining a history starts off simple and becomes more complex, the physical examination does as well. An organized physical examination proceeds in a step-by-step fashion and consists of the following: (Figure 3–8):

1. General inspection

2. Palpation (feeling)

3. Measuring motion

4. Neurologic examination

5. Examination of related areas

General Inspection

A great deal of information can be obtained by merely looking at someone and watching him or her move about. It doesn't take a medically trained eye to tell the difference between a person who is obviously out of shape, overweight and has poor posture and a person who is fit and trim with good posture (Figure 3–9). Likewise, if you have ever had or know someone who has had a severe case of low back pain, you know it is obvious to everyone around that something is wrong.

During the physical examination, the doctor inspects your spine both from the side and back while you stand. Since the spine should have a lazy S curve to it when viewed from the side, one of the first things your doctor looks for is an increase or decrease in these curves. Individuals with a spasm in their back muscles may have a straight, stiff spine, whereas a pregnant woman would likely have an increased curve in her lower back caused by her additional abdominal weight.

Viewed from the back, your spine should appear straight. Your shoulders and hips should also be level, balanced, and symmetric in appearance. If they are not, the

Figure 3–8 The components of a physical examination

Figure 3–9 "General Inspection"

spine may be curved (scoliosis). Your doctor should also measure each of your legs because a difference in their lengths may also account for an imbalance in the hip or shoulder area. A doctor examining the areas surrounding your spine will also be able to tell whether or not you have any obvious deformity or swelling, skin abnormalities or muscle atrophy.

Palpation

After a general inspection is performed, a doctor will palpate the bones, muscles and soft tissues of your spine to feel for tenderness, spasm and deformity. The spinous processes (bony prominences of the posterior aspect of the spine), as well as the interspinous ligaments between each spinous process, should be examined from your skull to your pelvis. Your doctor should feel for deformity and determine the precise areas that are painful to touch. The bones of your pelvis are also palpated. Your paraspinal, gluteal, thigh and abdominal muscles will also be examined for pain and spasm.

Figure 3–10   Palpation

Range of Motion

Your spine can move in a number of directions. Measuring the motion of your spine to determine if you are restricted in motion or if a certain motion is painful is another step in the physical examination of your spine. The movements of the spine are flexion, extension, lateral bending and rotation. To test flexion, you are required to bend over with your knees straight to see how close you can get your fingertips to the ground. Extension is bending backwards. Lateral bending and rotation should be comparable going each way (Figure 3–11). These motion tests are performed to evaluate any significant restriction in spinal motion.

Dysfunction of any of the components of your spine can cause painful or restricted motion. A problem with the bones or ligaments of your spine, muscle tightness or spasm, or sciatic nerve irritation can all affect the amount of motion of your spine.

The straight leg raise test (Figure 3–12) is one of the motion tests commonly used by physicians to evaluate your spine. To perform the straight leg raise test, begin by lying flat on your back. Keeping your legs straight, your doctor raises one of them into the air and measures the angle that your leg can be raised from the horizontal. A normal straight leg raise is 90 degrees or more.

Figure 3–11 Determining range of motion (left to right): flexion, extension, lateral bending, and rotation

Figure 3–12 The straight leg raise test

The motion measured by the straight leg raise test can be limited by a number of factors, including pain in your back, tightness in your hamstring muscles and irritation of your sciatic nerve. It is important to try to determine the limiting factor in performing this straight leg raise. If the restricting factor involves your back, low back pain will occur with the maneuver. If it is tight hamstrings, pain or tightness will be felt in the back of your upper leg or behind your knee when the test is performed. If the limiting factor is an irritated sciatic nerve, you will experience shooting pains into the involved leg because the straight leg raise test puts tension on that nerve.

Neurologic Examination

The sciatic nerve is a combination of several spinal nerves that exit the spinal column independently, merge into one large nerve and descend to the lower leg through your buttocks and thigh all the way to your foot (Figure 3–13). When your sciatic nerve is irritated, there may be tenderness along the course of the nerve. The area that the sciatic nerve travels through in the buttocks (the sciatic notch) can be palpated deep in the buttock between two bony prominences, one on your hip and the other on your pelvis. If your sciatic nerve is irritated (sciatica), then palpation of the sciatic notch will be painful. Also, if sciatica is present, the straight leg raise test will cause shooting pains along the course of the nerve into your foot because performing the test increases tension and pressure on the already irritated sciatic nerve.

SCIATIC NERVE

Figure 3–13   The sciatic nerve

Your doctor will also check your sciatic nerve by assessing the sensation, muscle function and reflexes in your leg. Additionally, the several spinal nerves that combined to form the sciatic nerve should each be individually tested. The three spinal nerves most affected in sciatica are the fourth lumbar (L4), fifth lumbar (L5), and first sacral (S1) nerves.

The L4 nerve exits your spine at the level of fourth lumbar vertebra, supplies sensation to the inside of your foot and is mainly responsible for the muscle that raises your ankle (anterior tibial muscle). It is also responsible for the knee jerk reflex.

The L5 nerve exits at the fifth lumbar vertebra, supplies sensation to the top of your foot and works the muscle that raises your big toe (extensor hallucis longus muscle).

The S1 nerve exits at the first sacral vertebra, supplies sensation to the outside of your foot, works the muscles that allow your ankle and foot to move downward (gastrocnemius and soleus muscles) and controls the ankle jerk reflex.

Examination of Related Areas

Although this book is concerned with back pain caused by problems in your back, you should remember that other areas of your body can refer pain to your back and may also need to be examined. Painful conditions, such as hip arthritis, may initially mimic back pain. Problems in your hips, knees or ankles can also affect your spine and cause back pain. In addition, stomach, intestinal, kidney, pelvis and other internal problems may manifest themselves as back pain (Figure 3–14).

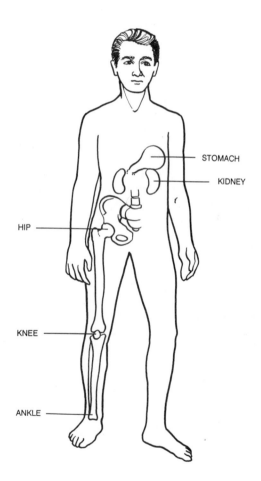

Figure 3–14 Examination of related areas

X-RAYS AND OTHER STUDIES

After completion of a history and a physical examination, your doctor may decide that it is appropriate to order X-rays and other studies to assist in an evaluation of your back pain. Regular X-rays are usually the initial test used to evaluate the bones of your back, just as they are used to evaluate the bones elsewhere in your body. Other X-ray studies, such as a computerized tomography, myelogram, bone scan or magnetic resonance imaging, are also sometimes used in an evaluation of back pain. Blood work is occasionally another component of the evaluative process for back pain. All of these tests, however, should complement — not replace — the history of your back pain and a thorough physical examination.

Depending on the history of your back pain and the results of your physical examination, your doctor may decide that it is not appropriate to order X-rays for you. On the other hand, your history and physical examination may indicate that extensive testing is required. The process and relative need for testing is illustrated by the following two examples:

1. A 10-year-old active boy falls off his slow-moving bike but continues to play all day and only complains the next day to his mother that he has a little pain in his back. At this time, it is probably not worth exposing this young boy to the unnecessary radiation of X-rays.

2. A previously healthy 20-year-old athlete injured her back two weeks ago and now has progressive pain in her back and legs with numbness and weakness in her legs. In this instance, extensive testing to determine the cause of this problem could be indicated.

X-rays

Regular X-rays are usually the initial study ordered in an evaluation of back problems. Most always, a minimum of two X-rays are obtained. One is a front-to-back view of your spine, and the other is a side view. Other X-ray views, such as oblique views, may also be taken to get a different view of the bones of your spine. X-rays of your spine will show if there is a problem with the bones of your spine, such as a fracture, arthritis, bone spurs or a curvature of the spine (Figure 3–15).

Computerized Tomography (CT) Scan

A CT scan is a special X-ray study that adds a three-dimensional effect to an X-ray evaluation of your spine (Figure 3–16). A CT scan provides your physician with a cross sectional view of your spine, rather than the front-to-back, side or oblique views produced by regular X-rays. The cross sectional view seen on a CT scan is the view you would have if you were able to see your spine from above. The level of your spine that is to be evaluated by a CT scan can be varied so that multiple cross sectional views are obtained.

Figure 3–15 An X-ray revealing a compression fracture

Figure 3–16 CT scan

A CT scan shows not only the bones of your spine, but also the soft tissues, such as the discs, the spinal cord and the nerves. A CT scan may be used in the evaluation of the bones of your spine because it provides a view different than regular X-rays, and therefore can be helpful in assessing fractures or arthritis. Because it gives multiple cross sectional views of your spine and the area that your spinal cord occupies, a CT scan is very helpful in determining if there is pressure on your spinal cord or nerves from an injured disc or from arthritis. A CT scan has about five times the radiation than that of a regular X-ray study of the spine.

Myelogram

A myelogram is an X-ray study done after a special dye is injected into the fluid surrounding your spinal cord and nerves (Figure 3–17). After the dye is injected into the spinal fluid, regular X-rays or a CT scan can be performed.

Normally the spinal fluid flows freely around the spinal cord up and down your spine from your brain (above) to your lower back (below). If pressure exists on your spinal cord or nerves, the spinal fluid will not flow freely. An X-ray taken after an injection of the dye will show an indentation on the spinal cord or nerves. A disc that has slipped, ruptured or herniated will cause pressure on the spinal cord and produce an indentation that can be seen on a myelogram study. The same thing can happen if there is a displaced fracture, a bone spur or a significant arthritis of the bones of your spine.

Figure 3–17   Myelogram

Bone Scan

A bone scan (Figure 3–18) is a study performed by injecting a radioactive labelled material into your bloodstream and then using a machine like a Geiger counter to measure the amount of this material absorbed in your bones. The material that is injected contains phosphorous, which is one of the minerals normally found in bone. When phosphorous is injected into your bloodstream, it is absorbed into the bone in small amounts. By adding a small amount of nondangerous radioactive phosphorous to this solution, the phosphorous that is taken up by the bones can then be measured by the Geiger counter. If there is an area in which bone is actively being made, such as a recent fracture that is healing, uptake of the phosphorous solution by that bone is much greater than in the surrounding bones. This process is shown by increased activity or uptake on the bone scan. In addition to a fracture, other bone processes that make or destroy bone will usually be apparent on a bone scan. Fractures, infections and arthritis will increase bone activity, whereas tumors may either increase or decrease activity.

Although bone scans do not provide the detail of regular X-rays, they do give a different type of information that may be valuable in the evaluation of back pain. A bone scan has about five times the radiation of a regular X-ray study of the spine.

Figure 3–18   Bone scan showing increased activity in L1 vertebra

Magnetic Resonance Imaging (MRI)

MRI is the most recently developed of the various types of studies used in the evaluation of the spine. The images created by MRI are made using magnetic fields that do not produce radiation exposure. MRI combines the benefits of regular x-rays and CT scans to provide a picture that shows not only the bones, but also the soft tissues (Figure 3–19). Accordingly, MRI results can be very valuable in helping to evaluate the structures of your back, especially pressure on your spinal cord from a disc injury, arthritis or bone spurs. At present, however, because it is a newer study and costs considerably more that

Figure 3–19   Magnetic resonance imaging showing a herniated disc

other types of X-ray tests, MRI is not as readily available to the back pain sufferer. MRI shows great promise, however, for the future in evaluating back disorders.

Blood Tests

In the evaluation of back pain, it may also be appropriate to order blood or other laboratory tests. Blood tests can show if an inflammatory arthritis, such as rheumatoid arthritis or ankylosing spondylitis, is present. Blood tests can also help indicate whether or not an infection is present. Blood or other laboratory tests can also provide valuable information to enable your doctor to determine if other problems, such as tumors or kidney infections, may be causing your back pain.

GETTING A SECOND OPINION

"Get a second opinion" is advice that is often easier given than acted upon. Whether or not you decide to pursue this course of action is entirely up to you. Whether or not you should feel the need to consider getting a second opinion depends on any number of factors. Do you have confidence in your doctor? Would a second opinion enhance your confidence in your doctor's advice? What are the risk factors involved in your doctor's advice? Obviously, the greater the risks, the greater your need to do all you can to make sure that you select the best course of action. And remember, the choice is yours and yours alone. Do you feel like you've been rushed into considering surgery by your doctor? Have you had a previous operation for the same condition? Has your doctor guaranteed the results from the proposed surgery? Has your doctor explained your situation to you in terms that you can understand? Do you believe you've been treated fairly?

If you decide to obtain a second opinion, it should be from a doctor who is at least as well qualified as the first. Once you've opted for a second opinion, however, you must decide what to do if the second opinion differs substantially from the first. We strongly recommend that you remember that you should not permit yourself to be rushed into a decision on what treatment you should adopt. Only in rare instances (paralysis or increasing loss of sensation or motor power) is time a crucial factor in your decision. So proceed cautiously—don't make a hasty decision.

4

FROM DIAGNOSIS TO THERAPY: HOW TO TREAT BACK PAIN

"Primum non nocere." *(First of all, do no harm.)*

– Hippocrates

The statistics on back pain present an extraordinarily bleak picture: over 10 million sufferers annually, over 100 million workdays lost every year, over 5 billion dollars in direct and indirect treatment costs and bouts of pain and intolerable anguish so seemingly countless as to give new meaning to the term "implausible." And yet, for all of the world's technological advances, for all of the evolutionary advances in the body of medical knowledge relating to pain, a simple fact remains: the mysteries of back pain often defy simple solutions. It is somewhat easier to explain why this is so than to accept the explanation. *At best, medicine is not an exact science.* If it were, surely a world in which the means were created for travel among the stars of the outer reaches of the universe would find a way to identify a foolproof method of treating (and preventing) back pain.

Since you have purchased this book and are reading this chapter, we assume that you have painfully discovered that considerable debate exists within the medical community on how to effectively treat back pain. This chapter presents an overview of the most typical approaches and means for treating back pain. For discussion purposes, the possible therapies are divided into two groups: nonsurgical and surgical.

NONSURGICAL THERAPIES

First, the good news. Your chances of not needing surgery to treat your back condition are excellent. Most back pain can be eliminated through one or a combination of any of the nonsurgical back therapies discussed in this section. In fact, the need for much of the back surgery currently conducted has been subject to considerable questioning. Now, the bad news. There are no guarantees — no treatment, surgical or nonsurgical, can guarantee elimination of your back pain.

Physicians have found that most of the nonsurgical therapies discussed in this section have a 60 to 70 percent chance of being successful. Which one should you use? This is something that you should discuss with your doctor. In fact, were you to check with several different physicians, it is likely that you would receive several different pieces of advice. Our advice to you is to try two or three of the nonsurgical treatment options. If your back pain persists after your nonsurgical efforts, it is then time to consider other alternatives.

Figure 4–1 The mysteries of back pain often defy simple solutions.

Bed Rest

Lying in bed (except for an occasional visit to the bathroom) is the most commonly prescribed treatment for back pain, particularly in the acute phase. Bed rest is frequently effective because it reduces the mechanical irritation of your spine and diminishes the level of inflammation in the area surrounding the irritation. As a result, nature (vis-à-vis bed rest) may enable you to become pain-free without any additional action on your part. There are at least two possible problems, however, with bed rest therapy. First, it doesn't work for everyone. In fact, some individuals find that their back pain is aggravated by lying down. Second, most individuals don't have the time or patience to spend two to three weeks in bed. All too clearly, they realize that whatever factor initially caused their back pain is likely to do so again in the not too distant future. Despite these potential problems, bed rest is the oldest, and possibly the most widely prescribed, therapy for treating back pain. (*Note:* Detailed guidelines for the most appropriate position for lying in bed for preventing back pain are presented in Chapter 6.)

Drug Therapy

Drug therapy is another commonly accepted therapy for treating back pain. The most widely used drug is aspirin. Aspirin serves as both a painkiller and an anti-inflammatory to reduce the effect of the actual injury. Most physicians recommend that you take the maximum dose (three aspirin every four hours) as soon as possible after the onset of your back pain. Other drugs which, in addition to aspirin, are classified as "painkillers" include aspirin-like drugs (e.g., Tylenol) and certain narcotics (e.g,. codeine, morphine, Demerol, Darvon and Percodan).

Muscle relaxants comprise the second category of drugs sometimes prescribed for the treatment of back pain. This type of drug is only available through a doctor's prescription. Among the well-known muscle relaxants are Flexoril, Valium, Norflex and Robaxin. Although such drugs have been known to help some individuals, most reputable physicians are reluctant to prescribe them for the treatment of back pain because the possible negative effects outweigh the possible benefits.

Figure 4–2 Aspirin is the drug used most often to treat back pain.

The third classification of drugs which are often used to treat back pain is anti-inflammatory medicine. Generally, this type of drug is recommended for individuals who need an anti-inflammatory but for whom aspirin has an undesirable side effect. A listing of anti-inflammatory drugs includes: Motrin, Indocin, Butazolidone, Clinoril, Feldene and Tolectin.

The precautions you should be aware of and the possible side effects for each type of drug used to treat back pain are presented in Table 4–1. Whatever the drug you are advised to take, we strongly recommend that you try to use the *lowest* effective dosage.

Spinal Manipulation

This method involves manipulating the spine, ostensibly to realign the joints of the spine, with particular attention given to the condition of the soft tissues of the back and to the level of muscle relaxation. In general, most manipulations are indirectly performed on the pain sufferer. The sufferer's head, shoulders and hips are twisted by someone in an attempt to realign the spine. Direct manipulation is conducted by applying pressure directly to the spinous processes of specific vertebrae.

The most common practitioners of spinal manipulation are chiropractors. In the United States, chiropractors generally enjoy wide popularity despite the fact that they are not licensed physicians per se. They cannot prescribe medications or perform surgical operations. Licensed physicians who regularly employ manipulation as a treatment therapy for back pain are known as osteopathic physicians.

Table 4–1 Drugs used to treat back pain

DRUGS	PURPOSE	POSSIBLE SIDE EFFECTS	PRECAUTIONS
Flexeril Norflex Norgesic Parafon Forte Robaxin Roboxisal Soma Valium	Prescription drugs for muscle spasms.	Blurred vision Dizziness Drowsiness Increased heart rate Lightheadedness Nausea	Caution should be taken with individuals who have a history of high blood pressure, heart disease, epilepsy, urinary problems or suicidal tendencies. In addition, these drugs should not be taken along with alcohol, tranquilizers or anti-depressant drugs.
Butazolidin Clinoril Feldene Indocin Meclomen Motrin Nalfon Naprosyn Tolectin	Prescription anti-inflammatory drugs.	Blurred vision Constipation Cramps Dizziness Ear problems Flatulence Fluid retention Headaches Heartburn Intestinal bleeding Nausea Nervousness Ringing in ears Vomiting	Caution should be taken with individuals who have a history of kidney or liver disease, bleeding problems or peptic ulcers. In addition, individuals who are physically incapacitated in some way should be particularly cautious.
Advil Aspirin Datril Tylenol	Non-prescription drugs for pain or inflammation.	Mild gastrointestinal problems *Nausea *Cramps *Dizziness *Headache *Heartburn *Intestinal bleeding *Ringing in ears	Caution should be taken with individuals who have a history of kidney or liver disease or bleeding problems or peptic ulcers.
Codeine Darvon Demerol Percocet Percodan Talwin Tylenol w/ Codeine Tylox Vicodin	Prescription drugs for pain.	Constipation Depression of breathing Dizziness Drug addiciton Lightheadedness Nausea Sudden drop in blood pressure Vomiting	Caution should be taken with individuals who have a history of irregular heartbeats or kidney and liver problems. In addition, individuals who are physically incapacitated in some way should be particularly cautious.

* NOTE: Effects unlikely with Tylenol or Datril

With regard to spinal manipulation, two questions arise: "Does it work?" and "What are the dangers attendant to manipulation?" The answer to the first question depends almost entirely on who you ask. There is obviously a lot of positive subjective opinion among many of the individuals who have undergone manipulation, or it wouldn't be as popular as it is. On the other hand, argue critics of this technique, there is no statistical evidence to support the claim that spinal manipulation produces a greater reduction in back pain than nature's own healing. In view of the potential dangers, however slight, these individuals conclude that the potential risks of spinal manipulation outweigh the possible gains. The primary risk is the danger that "jostling" the spine, discs and nerves can result in worsening your condition or cause a far more serious injury. However rare the risks, some individuals would prefer to wait for nature to take its course. Others prefer to try out their options as soon as possible. It is hoped that research which is currently being conducted on spinal manipulation therapy will provide more definitive information in the future about its usefulness.

Heat/Cold Therapy

Applying heat or cold to the area of your back that is painful (using an ice pack, heating pad or lamp) is one of the oldest and most useful methods for relieving muscle spasms. Neither heat nor cold has any curative effects, but each is often successful in relieving muscle spasms. Although heat and cold are opposites, they accomplish the same thing in treating back pain—they increase blood flow to the affected area. Heat involves a reflex mechanism that stimulates the attendant nerves. In turn, the blood vessels in the area to which heat is applied become dilated (expanded) so that more blood flows and the metabolism of the muscles in the area (including the one that is in spasm) is increased. The net result is that the spasm "relaxes."

Applying cold to the area is also effective. Whereas heat expands the blood vessels, cold constricts them. Cold is used following an acute injury to minimize bleeding in an injured area and to minimize swelling. And yet, after cold is used for a period of time, the constricted blood vessels fatigue, and then they relax and dilate. In the end, then, cold and heat have essentially the same effect. Because it is more comfortable, most people prefer heat to cold. In reality, though, cold is uncomfortable only for the first few minutes. Then the area becomes numb. A momentary burning sensation is usually experienced when cold is first applied, but it subsides quickly as the cold therapy is continued.

Two basic questions arise concerning the use of heat or cold as a therapy for treating back pain: "In what form should either be applied?" and "How often should the therapy be used?" Heat can be used in many forms. The simplest, least expensive ones have been found to be as effective as the more expensive methods. At home, you can use a hot water bottle, a heating pad or a water-heated towel to provide the heat. In general, wet heat has been found to be more successful for most people than dry heat. Wet or dry, you should apply the heat to your muscle spasm for approximately 20 to 30 minutes each session, two to four times a day. If you are particularly fortunate or resourceful, a hot tub is often an effective method for relieving a muscle spasm. Physicians will sometimes use deep heat as part of their treatment efforts for your back. Usually these efforts involve either diathermy or ultrasound. Diathermy uses a machine which, when applied to the area, produces a rapidly alternating electrical field that produces heat below the surface area of your skin by inducing movement in the molecules of your body's tissues. Ultrasound is the deepest form of heat therapy. The ultrasound waves, when applied to your skin where your pain is located, vibrate deep in your tissues, agitating the molecules in the tissues, and in turn causing them to produce heat in the affected area.

Cold is usually applied using an ice pack. Like heat, cold should be used two to four times a day. Ice packs should be applied to the affected area for 15 to 20 minutes at a time. A more effective way to use ice for cold therapy is to massage or rub the ice over the affected area. A technique that can be used for doing this is to freeze paper cups three-quarters filled with water. Then simply tear away just enough of the top portion of the cup to expose the ice and gently rub the skin over the affected area with it. Ice should be applied for approximately 30 seconds longer once the area being rubbed feels numb.

Massage

Like heat/cold therapy, massage is a method for treating muscle spasms that involves no risks and often provides immediate relief. Massage is passive exercise. Most massage treatments are applied painlessly by having someone rub or knead selected areas of your body. For most individuals, the process has psychological, as well as physiological, benefits. Psychologically, the stroking of our bodies has a soothing effect. Physiologically, massage stimulates the nervous system, which in turn elicits a response by your respiratory and circulatory systems. More blood is brought to the muscle in spasm because the blood vessels are dilated. Nourishment is delivered via the blood to the affected area, and more waste products are removed. The (desired) net result is that massage helps to relax muscles in spasm. Specific types of massage include home (nonprofessional) massage, professional massage, convective tissue massage and zone therapy. Although none of these forms has any documented curative powers, each seems to be an effective means of relieving back pain for some people.

Back Support Devices

A wide variety of braces, corsets and collars is currently on the market. Collectively, these devices purport to help relieve back pain by providing abdominal support or by supporting the spine. The better planned devices are designed for effective abdominal compression and for a slightly flexed lumbar spine. Lumbar flexion minimizes the degree to which the lumbar disc can bulge backwards, and it decreases some of the forces on the lumbar spine's posterior elements.

The question of whether or not these devices actually help has received an equivocal response. Although some back pain sufferers have indicated that the devices did in fact help them, many physicians suggest that wearing these devices might even worsen your condition. If you decide to pursue the use of one of these devices, we recommend that you proceed cautiously. You should wear one only after having undergone a thorough clinical examination by an experienced physician and a reasonable trial of less expensive therapy.

Traction

Traction involves some method for pulling the upper and lower parts of your body in opposite directions to ease your back pain. The machinery used to perform the traction ranges from weights, harnesses and pulleys to canvas slings (gravity lumbar reduction devices). Proponents of traction claim that it is an effective therapy because it allows you to "stretch" the various elements of the spine, thereby reducing the pressure on the affected nerves. Furthermore, they suggest that traction force can also be directed in a manner that helps to realign the joints of your back into their proper positions. This latter perceived characteristic is closely akin to what is supposed to occur with spinal manipulation. The protocol for applying traction varies from continuously for several hours to intermittent bouts for seconds or minutes. The amount of resistance (pull) typically used for traction for lower back pain ranges from 15 to as much as several hundred pounds. In the case of gravity lumbar reduction devices, your body's own weight is designed to do the work of the external force.

Considerable debate exists regarding whether or not traction is a useful form of therapy for back pain. Some physicians support its use, whereas others are adamantly against it. Whether to use traction or not is a decision that you should make carefully. Keep in mind that whatever the benefits of traction, they are short-lived. Once you stop being pulled, tugged and stretched, the elements of your spine will most likely go back to their old positions. One final note: We recommend that you religiously avoid all forms of inverted traction (e.g., inversion boots). No particular benefit exists because of your inverted position. On the contrary, an inverted position may cause microscopic bleeding in your eyes or brain.

Exercise

Exercises for back pain are designed to stretch and strengthen the muscles that support your spine, and to maintain flexibility in those muscles and other supporting structures. If you strengthen certain muscles and stretch certain ligaments, you will be better able to position your back so that the forces affecting your spine are better distributed, the pressure on your facet joints is reduced and the backward bulging of your discs is minimized. Remember that the strength of your spine can be attributed not to its bones, but to its musculature and the binding (harnessing) effects of its ligaments and connective tissues.

There is seemingly wide consensus on the value of exercise to both treat and prevent back pain. Obviously, the primary focus of exercising involves the prevention of back pain.

The use of exercises as a means for preventing back pain is discussed at length in Chapter 5 and Chapter 6. Chapter 5 presents a comprehensive overview of the

Figure 4–3   Many people agree that exercise can help treat and prevent back pain.

BackMate protocol—a system of exercises for stretching and strengthening the lower back which was developed and successfully tested at the United States Military Academy, West Point, New York. Chapter 6 includes a review of the traditional exercises used to develop the musculature supporting your back (stretching exercises, abdominal exercises and lower back exercises). Procedures for organizing an exercise program to prevent back pain are also presented in Chapter 6.

Invasive Methods

Invasive methods for treating back pain involve techniques in which your body is invaded (entered) in some way. Acupuncture, trigger point injections, cortisone and novocaine injections and chemonucleolysis are the most common types of invasive methods. Although each of the techniques described in this section have brought relief to some individuals, we recommend that you remember that every invasive medical procedure carries some degree of medical risk.

Acupuncture. Acupuncture has evolved out of three thousand years of Chinese culture and history, and it entails placing thin needles at specific points of your body in order to dull or mask your back pain. The placement of the needles is arranged along lines of energy, called meridians, that run up, down and around your body, and have purportedly been mapped out over thousands of years by Chinese doctors. In some instances, the needles are supplemented by a low-voltage electrical current. Acupuncture has produced equivocal results. Some individuals swear by its effectiveness, while others claim not to have been helped by the procedure. In support of the former conclusion, some studies have indicated that acupuncture stimulates your body's production of endorphins, thereby relieving your back pain.

Trigger Point Injections. Trigger point treatment involves injecting a local anesthetic into specific points that have been identified as producing pain at other sites in your back. Stimulating the trigger points in your back (unduly sensitive muscle areas) by means of injections is believed to somehow break up the pain cycle in your back. A considerable degree of uncertainty surrounds this method of back treatment. Like acupuncture, the results are mixed—it works well for some, and not at all for others. In addition, in some instances, a simple saline solution or simply needling the trigger point without injecting anything at all has been found to be as successful in treating back pain as an actual injection.

Cortisone and Novocaine Injections. Whereas acupuncture and trigger point injections are basically localized treatments, injecting cortisone and novocaine often involves painfully deep injections. Cortisone is injected in hopes of halting local inflammation. Cortisone can also be used for trigger point injections. Novocaine is an anesthetic that is injected in an attempt to interrupt the cycle of pain between the local pain and a secondary muscle spasm. In general, cortisone and novocaine injections have not been found to be more effective than milder therapies and in some instances have been found to be less effective.

Chemonucleolysis. Chemonucleolysis is a nonsurgical method for treating herniated or bulging discs. It involves injecting an enzyme, chymopapain, into the center portion of an injured disc. The enzyme, once injected, dissolves the nucleus (disc center) only, without affecting the adjacent outer portion of the disc, the nerves, the muscles and the ligaments. Dissolving the nucleus has been found to reduce the pressure (and thereby the pain) on the nerves near the disc. It should work better for a bulging disc than a herniated disc, where fragments of the disc may be within the spinal canal. The entire procedure for performing chemonucleolysis (from start to finish) takes about an hour and requires approximately one to five days of hospitalization afterwards. This therapy has been found to be somewhat safer than surgery, although certainly not risk-free, as very serious allergic reactions to the enzyme have occurred. Its success rate is comparable to other nonsurgical techniques.

Psychological Treatments

Few people realize just how closely their bodies and minds are intertwined. Each of us is, after all, just one organism. Studies have shown that specific psychologically focused therapies can be effective in treating back pain in certain instances. In general, these therapies fall into two groups. The first category involves efforts to relieve tension. If you relieve tension, you decrease the amount of muscular activity. When your muscle is tense, it is contracted. This contraction affects your nerves as well. Tension involves contraction, which in turn results in fatigue and pain because your nerves become electrically irritated. Eventually, you may experience excessive nervous tension, as well as excessive muscular tension. Too much tension can lead to back pain. Controlling your level of tension is essentially a function of learning to relax. It should be noted that relaxation is the opposite of movement. Relaxation is reflected by a reduction or a complete absence of muscular activity in your voluntary muscles. A number of effective techniques for learning how to relax have been developed, including progressive relaxation, mind-to-muscle relaxation, meditation, autogenic training, breathing training and visualization.

he second group of psychologically focused therapies involves techniques designed to enable you to "control" and "manage" your pain. Somewhat similar to the aforementioned relaxation techniques, these methods also focus on reducing the amount of tension you have. In addition, they attempt to change the way you perceive pain so that you are better prepared to deal with your pain, if necessary. Unfortunately, there are no guarantees that everyone will live a pain-free life. Those who have pain must learn to live with it. Learning how to gain control over your pain and your attendant emotions can be an invaluable action on your part. There are a number of diverse "control-and-manage" pain therapies, including biofeedback, hypnosis, progressive relaxation, visualization and behavioral analysis.

Back Pain Schools/Pain Clinics

A relatively recent development in the search to identify an effective means of treating back pain has been the establishment of organizations known generally as back pain schools or pain clinics. These organizations combine education with treatment within a setting of professional expertise and human understanding. Participation in the programs offered by these groups is designed to allow back pain sufferers to meet each other in a supportive and positive way. The treatment programs in these schools focus on educating you to accept responsibility for caring for your back, training you in the proper techniques for protecting your back and teaching you how to deal safely with the daily demands of your work and life. By offering the collective expertise of a diverse faculty of specialists and experts on back care, these clinics have been found to be a reasonable, effective, nonsurgical means of treating pain. In many instances they have proven to be more successful than other nonsurgical methods.

BackMate

BackMate is a treatment therapy that involves performing stretching and strengthening exercises using an apparatus called a BackMate. Conceived, designed and tested by two faculty members at the United States Military Academy, BackMate has been found to be a highly effective means for treating back pain. The BackMate program not only relieves back pain but, more importantly, it diminishes the chances of recurring back pain when performed systematically. Initially tested successfully on over 200 members of the USMA community (cadets, staff, faculty and dependents), BackMate is currently being evaluated in two major research studies — one involving Pepsi Cola executives at Pepsi Cola's worldwide headquarters, and one using chronic back pain patients at the H.E.A.R.T. Clinic of the New York Medical College. The BackMate program dismisses the idea that it is mandatory that back pain sufferers wait until their back pain diminishes before attempting to deal with it by exercising. Rather, relief from your pain is not only desirable, but possible. Initial studies suggest that BackMate therapy is a highly effective method for efficiently and safely treating back pain — particularly chronic pain in individuals who have unsuccessfully tried other nonsurgical techniques. A more comprehensive explanation of BackMate is presented in Chapter 5.

SURGICAL THERAPIES

Surgery serves a useful, but limited, function in treating back pain. In the vast majority of cases in which individuals suffer from back pain, surgery is not only unnecessary, but useless. There are only a few times when back surgery is essential. One is when pressure on a nerve must be diminished to relieve unmanageable pain. Another is when progressive nerve damage and paralysis must be halted. A third time is when there is painful motion in the spinal column that must be stopped to prevent recurrence of pain. There are also other, unusual circumstances in which your back pain may not be relieved within a *reasonable* period of time using nonsurgical therapies, and surgery is warranted. Whatever the problem is, though, it should have been present long enough to assume that nature alone is not going to treat it, and, in addition, nonsurgical therapies must have been tried and been unsuccessful. Finally, reasonable evidence should exist that surgery will correct, eliminate or improve your condition. Although no simple equation exists to give you an answer about whether or not you should have surgery, we strongly recommend that you adhere to the following advice: "If the risks involved in your surgery are high and the odds it will help are, at least in your opinion, low, it shouldn't be done."

The primary task of your physician, with regard to the question of whether or not you should have surgery, is to ensure that you are given sufficient information to make an informed decision. Cold statistics are one thing; your quality of life is quite another. The better informed you are, the more likely you will make a decision that is appropriate to *your* situation.

Once you and your physician have reached the decision that surgery is the best course of action for you, the type of surgery performed depends entirely on your condition. These procedures range from laminectomy (disc excision) to salvage back surgery (multiple back operations).

Laminectomy

The most common surgical procedure for back pain is a laminectomy. A laminectomy involves making a small opening in the lamina (the bone that is part of the vertebra which covers the affected level of the spinal canal). Once your physician can get at the slipped or herniated disc material that is pressing on the nerve root, it is removed. Any loose fragments within the space between the vertebrae or within the disc are also removed to prevent the possibility of the recurrence of pain. The operation, conducted with the patient under full anesthesia, normally takes anywhere from 30 to 90 minutes in the average-sized individual. Following surgery, the hospitalization period usually lasts from three to four days. After your discharge from the hospital, you should be able to resume full-time work in approximately three to four weeks. Full recovery (the operation is fully forgotten) usually takes about six months. The success rate for this type of surgical therapy is often as high as 90 percent.

Spinal Fusion

Spinal fusion, a special type of back surgery, is an operation in which bone from somewhere else in your body, or from a donor's body, is grafted onto living bone in your back. Eventually the grafted bone in your body will be replaced by living bone produced by your body. In the meantime, you have made a strong, stable union between two or more vertebrae (the bones selected for fusion). This stable union obviously reduces the motion at that particular segment of your spine. Any pain that had previously been produced or irritated by the excessive motion that existed will subside. The success rate of spinal fusion operations has not been found to be above the host of nonsurgical therapies discussed previously. For that reason, the incidence of spinal fusions has decreased dramatically in recent years. Except in instances in which the likely benefits of a spinal fusion are well-documented (e.g., following a severe spinal fracture in which the joints between the vertebrae are so severely injured that the stability of your spine is in question), the possible negative complications from a spinal fusion are too extensive to warrant such an operation.

Surgery to Relieve Spinal Stenosis

Spinal stenosis is a condition in which the space in your spinal canal is not big enough. This condition can be congenital. More often, though, it is the result of arthritis and bone spurs in your vertebral bodies or facet joints that cause narrowing of the spinal canal. Stenosis can also be caused by a degenerative or a herniated disc. The surgical procedure for this condition involves removing any and all structures that are impinging on the nerves within the spinal canal. If the need for this operation is confirmed beforehand by radiographic studies (myelogram or a CAT scan), the operation is usually successful.

Surgery to Treat Infections

Infections of the spine can be quite painful. Although antibiotics alone can often eliminate such infections, in some instances surgery may be necessary to treat them. In these cases, surgery is performed to drain the infection and to remove enough of the soft tissue and bone to cure the infection while maintaining as much of the spine as possible. A thorough cleansing of the area with a sterile solution containing antibiotics is also done to prevent recurrence of the infection. In some cases, depending upon how much of the bone had to be removed, a bone graft may subsequently be required to fuse and reconstruct the spine.

Surgery to Remove Tumors

The decision on whether or not to surgically remove a tumor must be made taking several factors into account. Can it be treated with chemotherapy or radiation? Is it benign or malignant? Did it originate in your spine, or has it migrated from elsewhere in your body? What are the risks involved in surgery for this specific tumor? What are the probable outcomes of both performing and not performing this surgery?

In general, the procedures of this type of surgery are similar to those for surgery to treat infections. Because the surgeon has to eliminate all of the tumor *plus* an appropriate margin of normal spine adjacent to the tumor, the surgical risks and skills needed to perform the operation successfully are substantially higher when operating to remove a tumor than for treating a spinal infection. The likelihood of needing a bone graft or other type of spinal replacement device or material to rebuild the spine after this operation is also increased.

Surgery to Treat Injuries

Moderate fractures of your spine tend to heal without severe pain. Surgery for spinal fractures depends to some extent on whether the fracture is old or recent. An old fracture probably will not require surgery unless severe pain is present and the pain can be reasonably attributed to the fracture. In this instance, your physician would probably immobilize you in a brace or body cast. If your pain decreases, a spinal fusion operation would probably help. Whether or not surgery would be required for a recent fracture depends on the extent of any vertebrae damage. If your vertebrae were extensively damaged, especially in your lower spine, you probably would undergo an operation in which stainless steel rods would be implanted next to your spine. Attached to your normal spine above and below your injury, these rods would help hold your spine in place while it heals. On the other hand, injuries such as mild compression fractures, expecially in the more stable area of the spine like the thoracic vertebrae, may require no more treatment than restricting the movement of the affected area while your fracture heals.

Surgery to Interrupt Your Nervous System

There are three surgical procedures designed to interrupt your nervous system. In each, an operation is performed to "inhibit" your pain by surgically cutting a specific pain pathway. The rationale is that the sensation of pain cannot be transmitted to your brain if the pain pathway has been severed. In a procedure called a *tractotomy*, a localized segment of your spinal thalamic tract is cut at the site where the sensory part of the affected nerves from your back and limbs enter your spinal cord. In a procedure called a *rhizotomy*, the nerves around the affected intervertebral joints are destroyed in an attempt to "deaden" the pain perceived to be emanating from these joints. Neither a tractotomy nor a rhizotomy has been found to be particularly successful. As a result, these procedures rarely are performed nowadays. In a procedure called a *cordotomy*, the pain pathways in the upper thoracic or cervical spinal cord are severed. This operation is only performed when a terminally ill cancer patient has severe, localized pain in one area of the body (such as one leg) and has a limited life expectancy.

Salvage Back Surgery

Salvage back surgery is surgery that is performed on someone who has already had two or more operations for back pain. Numerous studies suggest that additional surgical operations often have decreasing chances of success. As a result, except in those extremely rare circumstances when multiple back operations are warranted, you should be very cautious before undergoing surgery again.

THE NEXT STEP

The first four chapters of this book examined the basics of back pain: an anatomical overview of your back; the causes of back pain; how your doctor diagnoses and evaluates your back pain; and the most common nonsurgical and surgical therapies for treating back pain. Chapter 5 presents a discussion of the BackMate protocol.

5

WORKING TOGETHER: THE BACKMATE PROTOCOL

"It's a funny thing about life; if you refuse to accept anything but the best, you often get it."

– Somerset Maugham

To claim that back pain sufferers are constantly bombarded by a diverse array of new products and medical procedures, each promising to be a cure-all for back pain, would be a vast understatement. As we've stated several times previously in this book, there simply are no legitimate guarantees that product X or treatment procedure Y will successfully correct your back condition. Anyone who states otherwise should be viewed with a substantial degree of skepticism. Having reiterated that point, we'd like to share with you (for the first time ever in public print) information on a treatment program that has recently been developed at West Point, New York, which has been extraordinarily effective in treating back pain – the BackMate protocol.

Attempting to explain a new technique that apparently works better than any other nonsurgical therapy currently in use without sounding like a snake oil salesman or the proverbial used car salesman is, at best, a difficult task. We ask you to keep an open mind and remember that the procedures described in the following sections of this chapter were extensively tested on members of the West Point community – all of whom had unsuccessfully tried a variety of therapies for treating their back pain. The results of those tests provide the optimistic basis for this chapter.

WHAT IS BACKMATE?

BackMate is an exercise apparatus that enables your hamstring and lower back muscles to be stretched effectively and your lower back and buttock muscles to be strengthened safely and efficiently. In the BackMate protocol, individuals suffering from back pain lie flat on their back on the BackMate with their hips secured to the device in order to stabilize their back and pelvis. Using a training partner, each individual performs a series of exercises designed to stretch and strengthen the legs and lower back.

BackMate was initially conceived as a device to provide temporary relief by stretching the lower back. At the time, the alternatives for stretching the back were not appropriate for most individuals. Hanging by a bar, with your weight suspended from the bar, is one way to pull your body in opposite directions. However, this method is painfully ineffective for someone who doesn't have short arms, a reasonable amount of shoulder strength and a body type that is not in the least bit bottom-heavy. Another way to stretch your lower back is to use one of the wide variety of harnesses, pulleys and canvas slings designed for that purpose. At best, these devices offer an awkward, sometimes expensive, often ineffective approach to relieving your back pain. A third technique for stretching your back that was very popular several years ago involved the use of inversion or gravity boots. No upper body strength was required. All you had to do was put the boots on and hang upside down in an inverted position. Doctors soon discovered that there was no advantage in being in the inverted position. On the contrary, assuming an inverted position may produce microscopic bleeding in your eyes or brain. Another means commonly advanced to stretch your lower back muscles was to perform one or more stretching exercises that are supposed to accomplish that goal. The obvious difficulty in this alternative is that many individuals are not able (for whatever reason — lack of flexibility, muscular fitness or motor skill) to do these exercises when they're *not* in deep pain, let alone when they're suffering.

BackMate was developed partially in response to the shortcomings in the existing methods for stretching your lower back. The developers of BackMate concluded that your lower back muscles could be easily and safely stretched if you lay flat on your back with your pelvis and hips stabilized and had someone exert a moderate force on your legs in the direction of your head. At all times during the exercise, you are required to keep your knees locked (legs straight). Not surprisingly, individuals whose lower back muscles are stretched in this manner often experience immediate relief from their back pain.

The temporary nature of the relief provided by the stretching exercises encouraged the developers of BackMate to search for a method of preventing recurrence of back pain. This search led these researchers to the same dead ends encountered by all the others who had previously attempted to identify an acceptable method of treating back pain. Whereas only 60 to 70 percent of back pain sufferers could be successfully treated by nonsurgical means, surgical therapies could raise the success rate to 90 percent in certain instances. This is not a very impressive success rate, especially where nonsurgical procedures are concerned.

The individuals who developed the BackMate protocol found numerous limitations in the existing therapeutic options available to back pain sufferers. The primary one was the *invalid mentality* they inspired in individuals suffering from back pain: If you get hurt, lie down and let nature perform its healing "magic" on you. Once the pain has subsided, you should do a series of exercises designed to prevent the recurrence of your pain. If the exercises cause you discomfort (and they often do), refrain from performing them until the discomfort disappears. In the meantime, wait for the next inevitable bout of excruciating back pain. And then the cycle can begin anew. The back pain sufferers who—for whatever reason—couldn't be helped by these methodologies for treating back pain presented another shortcoming in the existing knowledge base. A nonexclusive listing of other deficiencies that can be identified in some of the traditional therapies for treating back pain includes: the risk factor, cost, ease of application and temporal nature of beneficial effects.

The essence of the BackMate protocol—the strengthening phase—was subsequently discovered during an extensive review of the literature concerning which exercises could be performed to treat and prevent back pain. Although several researchers had recommended that back pain sufferers perform exercises to strengthen their lower back muscles, the exercises that they recommended simply were culled from a pool of traditionally performed exercises. None of these exercise protocols properly isolated the muscles of the lower back so that these muscles could be worked in a direct, intense manner. None placed a specific, full-range-of-movement demand on the musculature of the lower back. This shortcoming is not surprising when you remember that within the world of athletics—an arena of individuals who frequently spend considerable time and effort developing their level of muscular fitness—no exercises exist that will safely and effectively develop the musculature of the lower back. Although there are exercises that will strengthen your back, they don't achieve this goal in a safe, effective, efficient manner.

At the United States Military Academy, there has always been an uncompromising institutional emphasis on providing all cadets with the most appropriate advice possible with regard to taking care of their bodies physically. Accordingly, the research conducted to treat and eliminate back pain in the Corps of Cadets was extensive. The developers of BackMate were well aware of the requirements of the exercises they were looking for to strengthen the muscles of the lower back. They subsequently discovered that once you've performed the stretching exercises on the BackMate, you can isolate and work your lower back and buttock muscles in a very intense manner if you keep your knees locked while exerting a downward force against moderate resistance provided by a training partner. Your partner allows you to continue to move your legs against this resistance from a point slightly more than perpendicular to the ground (or less if you are unable to reach that point because of a lack of hamstring flexibility) to a point approximately 45 degrees from the ground (past this point you would hyperextend your back and put undesirable pressure on the affected structures of your spine). Testing their theory that strengthening the lower back muscles would both help treat back pain and prevent its recurrence confirmed their hypothesis. Over 200 members of the West Point community and the surrounding area (including several physicians) engaged in the BackMate protocol over a period of two years. In every instance, substantial improvement in the level of back pain was reported by the sufferer. Currently, two highly structured research studies on the effects of BackMate are being conducted — one with back pain patients at the New York College of Medicine, and one involving Pepsi Cola executives at their worldwide headquarters.

HOW DOES BACKMATE WORK?

The world of medicine is fraught with a sense of the unknown. Physicians often have a good idea about how or why something occurs, but are unable to state how or why it occurs with total accuracy. Why, for example, does aspirin affect one individual one way and another individual a different way? Why do some people get cancer and others who have led a similar lifestyle don't? How can one set of parents have four offspring who differ substantially in appearance from each other? How can an individual who has led an active, health-conscious life suffer a heart attack, and a sedentary individual with terrible eating habits avoid a heart attack? And so on. A listing of examples of the many unknowns of medicine and the human body is almost endless.

Pain — specifically back pain — is another of the mysteries of medicine. Why do some people react in an entirely different way to pain than others? Why are some people more pain-sensitive than others? Why do some people have a high threshold for pain and not others? Why do individuals with apparently the same kind of pain respond differently to the same therapy? Why will a certain therapy work for one person and not another? And so on.

Over the years a number of theories have been advanced by members of the medical community to explain the phenomenon of pain, specifically, how it's initiated and why it subsides. Unfortunately, the discussion over the causes and proper treatment of pain continues. The mere fact that there is as much discussion as there is regarding the treatment of back pain confirms the fact that considerable disagreement over this matter still exists.

Given the enigmas of pain, it is not difficult to accept the fact that all explanations of why a specific therapy controls pain involve some theory and assumption. Explaining why BackMate is such an effective means for treating back pain is no different. We know it works very well for most people. We think we know exactly how it works for you, but no explanation can give full account of the intricacies of pain reduction.

The key to the effectiveness of the BackMate protocol is the ability of the BackMate exercises to break the cycles of pain affecting your back. The consequences of fully stretching your hamstring and lower back muscles and properly strengthening your buttock and lumbar muscles has been shown to effectively stop the cycle of pain. The critical question is: How does this occur?

Unlike conventional back exercises, the use of a belt while using BackMate provides adequate stabilization of your pelvis and optimum isolation of your lumbar muscles during the exercises. In addition, by lying on the flat surface of the Back-Mate, you further reduce unwanted motion during the exercises and achieve additional stabilization of your pelvis. The high level of pelvic stabilization permits you to be able to focus on stretching your lumbar and hamstring muscles. This, in turn, produces a gapping of the posterior structures (facets, soft tissue) in your lumbar region, which reduces the pressure on your spinal nerve endings. A decrease in this pressure tends to promote a corresponding decrease in back pain. BackMate stretching exercises also appear to stimulate the local mechanoreceptors to produce localized secretions of endorphins and enkephalins, which further aids in pain reduction.

Performing the BackMate stretching exercises also produces a vigorous contraction of your hamstring and lumbar spine muscles. This contraction allows each of these muscle groups to relax reflexively. This relaxation permits a greater range of motion in your back and lower extremities. This increased level of mobility in your back and flexibility in your hamstrings enable you to move through a greater range of movements without experiencing typical mechanical lower back discomfort.

The BackMate protocol has several additional consequences that collectively tend to reduce your level of back pain. The isolated contraction of your lumbar muscles that occurs during both the stretching and the strengthening phases of BackMate stimulates an increase in local circulation in your lower back and the removal of some of the toxic metabolites that have accumulated in these muscles from lack of use. Finally, and perhaps most importantly, strengthening the postural muscles in your lower back enables these muscles to sustain themselves longer without the buildup of toxic metabolites brought on by chronic fatigue. Stronger lower back muscles are more capable of permitting you to maintain a proper body alignment. In addition, stronger lower back muscles (all other factors being equal) are less susceptible to being injured and more capable of withstanding the debilitating effects of outside forces on your body.

THE BACKMATE PRESCRIPTION

There are a number of items to consider when deciding when it would be appropriate to see a doctor. Your sense of urgency to each and your response to each are personal matters. Before undergoing the BackMate protocol, however, we strongly recommend that you see your physician to ensure that there is no medical reason (e.g., infection, tumor) to preclude doing BackMate exercises. This section presents detailed, illustrated instructions on how to perform the BackMate protocol.

Preliminary Instructions

1. Open your BackMate and place it flat on the floor with the restraining strap unbuckled (Figure 5–1).

2. Lie flat on your back on the Back-Mate so that your spine is over the padded portion of the board (Figure 5–2). For additional comfort, you may want to place a towel or pillow under your head.

3. Next, close the restraining strap buckle and pull the straps on each side of the buckle so that the strap fits snugly across your hips. (For added comfort you may want to place a towel between you and the strap).

4. The BackMate conditioning/strengthening program consists of two parts. The first part is designed to stretch your back and leg muscles, whereas the second part is designed to strengthen your lower back muscles. The starting position is the same for both portions of the BackMate program.

Figure 5–1   The BackMate

Figure 5–2 Lie flat on your back on the BackMate, close the restraining strap buckle and pull the straps until the strap fits snugly across your hips.

Starting Position

1. The BackMate program incorporates a Training Partner (TP), to provide an intelligent resistance that is necessary to perform the stretching and strengthening exercises properly.

2. To assume the starting position for the BackMate program, your TP stands with one foot on the BackMate to hold it down. The TP then stoops down and grasps each of your legs at the ankle and raises your legs, with your knees locked, until your legs form a 90 degree angle with the floor, or as close to 90 degrees as possible (Figure 5–3). Less flexible people are often not able to attain a 90 degree starting position. You should attempt to start both parts of the exercise, however, as close to the 90 degree starting position as you can without discomfort.

3. It is very important that you keep your legs straight and your knees locked throughout the BackMate program and that you let your TP control your legs. Do not make any effort to move or hold up your legs. If your TP feels that you are helping to move or hold your legs up, he or she should remind you to relax and let your TP do the work. (Let your TP " have your legs.")

4. You are now ready to begin the BackMate program.

Figure 5–3 Your training partner raises your legs until they form a 90 degree angle with the floor.

Stretching Your Lower Back and Legs

1. Your TP stretches your lower back muscles and the hamstring muscles of your legs by gently pushing your legs from the starting position toward your head (with your knees locked), to the extent that the stretching is effective but not too uncomfortable (Figure 5–4). Your TP then brings your legs back to the

starting position. Six to eight repetitions of stretching should be completed before and after each strengthening workout session on your BackMate.

2. If you are relatively inflexible, some degree of discomfort may be experienced in the area behind your knees. Such discomfort is the result of stretching the hamstring muscle at its point of insertion (an added benefit of the BackMate program). This discomfort should subside over a period of time as you continue the stretching portion of the BackMate program. After several exercise sessions with your BackMate, this discomfort should disappear as you increase your flexibility.

3. As your flexibility increases, you will get closer to assuming the 90 degree starting position if you were not able to do so at the start of your program. Increased flexibility will also enable your TP to move your legs farther from the starting position toward your head while you are stretching.

4. After stretching, you are ready for the strengthening portion of the exercise.

Figure 5–4   Your training partner gently pushes your legs toward your head.

Strengthening Your Lower Back

1. Your TP helps you strengthen your back by providing an intelligent resistance when you move your legs from the starting position toward the floor. The TP does this by maintaining the same grip on your ankles that was used during the stretching part of the exercise. The TP controls the downward movement of your legs, allowing them to move in a steady, smooth pattern (Figure 5–5).

2. Your TP should provide the resistance necessary so it takes you about three to four seconds to move your legs from the starting position to a position at

about the knee level of your TP. Your TP should pay attention to proper back care techniques when providing resistance for you, especially if you are fairly strong. (*Note:* Refer to Chapter 6.)

3. Your TP then raises your legs again (relax and let the TP do the work), attempting this time to take your legs to a point slightly farther back than the previous starting position. At that starting point, you perform another repetition of the exercise.

4. For maximum results you should perform 8 to 12 repetitions of the strengthening portion of the exercise.

5. At all times during the stretching and strengthening portion of the exercise, you should try to keep your knees locked. This will permit maximum stretching for both the hamstring and lower back muscles during the stretching phase and maximum strengthening of the lower back and buttock muscles during the strengthening phase.

Figure 5–5 Your training partner provides resistance as you move your legs from the starting position toward the floor, until they are at about the level of your training partner's knees.

Frequency of Exercise

1. If you are currently suffering from lower back pain when you obtain your Back-Mate, you should perform one session as described previously as soon as possible. This should provide immediate relief.

2. You should then use your BackMate on a daily basis unless your pain reoccurs within 24 hours. If the pain returns before your next scheduled workout, your BackMate should be used as soon as possible to relieve pain.

3. Once your back pain subsides for 24 hours or more, you should try to establish a back maintenance program that includes using your BackMate as
   described earlier at least three times per week. Additional flexibility exercises
   as described in Chapter 6 can be used to augment the BackMate exercises.

WHY BACKMATE?*

The answer to the question, "Why BackMate?" is fairly basic: "No one should
needlessly suffer back pain." We have found the BackMate program to be a very
successful method for eliminating back pain and preventing its recurrence in
individuals whose condition is due to muscular problems, and reducing back pain to
a much more manageable level in individuals whose back pain is the result of a
structural problem. Table 5–1 presents a general comparative overview of BackMate
and traditional nonsurgical and surgical therapies.

*Note: Additional information on the BackMate can be obtained by contacting:

LIFEMATES
9501 West Devon Avenue   Suite 203
Rosemont, IL 60018
1-800-442-4447 / 312-825-0824

Table 5-1 A comparison of the benefits and costs between BackMate® and traditional nonsurgical and surgical therapies

BENEFITS/COST	BACKMATE	TRADITIONAL NON-SURGICAL THERAPIES	TRADITIONAL SURGICAL THERAPIES
CHANCES OF SUCCESS IN TREATING PAIN	90 + %	60–70%	90%
SAFETY FACTOR— EXTENT OF RISKS	Very safe; minimal risk	Depending on the therapy, reasonably safe; some are more risky than others	Almost always safe, but the risks associated with back surgery can be great
CHANCE OF PROVIDING IMMEDIATE RELIEF	Very good	2–3 weeks on the average	Takes at least one month, sometimes longer
EASE OF APPLICATION	Very easy, except that a training partner is needed	Ranges from very easy (bed rest) to somewhat difficult (invasive treatment)	Not easy; formidable in some instances
TIME INVOLVED	Less than 2 minutes per day	Ranges from hours to weeks	Considerable; recovery can take months
EXPENSE INVOLVED	Less than $200	Ranges from no expense at all to somewhat expensive	Very expensive
LOCATION OF TREATMENT	Anywhere— home, work, leisure	Specific to the treatment	Hospital or doctor's office
RESPONSIBILITY FOR TREATMENT	Your own	Specific to the treatment	Doctor

6

PREVENTING BACK PAIN: ADVICE FOR DAILY LIVING

"To take what there is, and use it, without waiting forever in vain for the preconceived—to dig deep into the actual and get something out of that—this doubtless is the right way to live."

—Henry James

This chapter is for people at various stages of back pain or recovery from it. It presents basic guidelines on how to take care of your back properly after you've recovered from a bout of back pain and want to avoid a recurrence. It is also for you to consult when your pain is in the process of subsiding and you want to do whatever is feasible to expedite the process. Finally, it offers general suggestions to individuals who have never had back pain on what to do to maximize their chances of avoiding it.

As you can readily see, almost everyone can identify with one of the three aforementioned categories. Either you've had back pain in the past and would like to avoid another bout in the future, you currently have back pain and want to get rid of it as painlessly and as quickly as possible, or you've never had back pain and want to continue in that fortunate state for the foreseeable future. Our advice to each person is the same: "Identify an appropriate plan for your daily living to enable you to achieve your goal and follow your plan." In other words, develop a strategic plan for your life. The critical elements of such a plan are the same for all three categories of individuals. First, learn what makes good sense concerning your back as you perform all your customary daily tasks. Second, reduce the load that your spine must carry around and your back muscles must support by shedding excess poundage. Third, engage in a properly designed exercise program to stretch and strengthen your back muscles and the muscles supporting your back. Fourth, if you are a woman, be aware of the fact that there are some back-related problems that only women have. You should design your "strategic" plan for daily living accordingly.

GOOD SENSE REGARDING CUSTOMARY TASKS

If you are serious about avoiding back pain, you must take some care in how you go about performing your "normal" tasks. Biomechanically, there is a proper way that these activities should be performed if you wish to keep the stresses on your lower spine and back muscles to a minimum. Increasing the stresses can result in a corresponding increase in the likelihood that you will encounter back pain at some point in your life. Accordingly, you should adhere as closely as possible to steps that will minimize stress on your lower spine, whatever the task.

Posture

Your first step in preventing back pain is to maintain good posture in all of your body's positions. Failure to do so will place undesirable stress on your back. Understanding a simple law of physics can explain why this is so. This law states that when a force is applied to a curved structure, the greatest stress is applied on the inner (concave)

Figure 6–1   You must take some care as you perform the tasks that are normal in your life.

side of the curve. As a result, the greater the curve in your spine, the more uneven the amount of pressure over your spine, with the largest force concentrated at the apex of the curve. In turn, this circumstance then results in excessive wear on your intervertebral joints at the apex of the curve of your spine. This excessive wear may subsequently cause your back to be affected earlier than normal by degenerative changes or wear-and-tear factors.

It is not difficult to comprehend why individuals with good posture are less likely to suffer back pain or be injured that individuals with poor posture. Individuals with poor posture put too much strain on their backs by localizing too much of the stress on one area of their spine. Individuals with good posture are able to distribute more of the forces being applied to their spine throughout their entire spine.

Good posture is essential whether you're standing, sitting, bending over, rising up, sleeping or performing any of your many daily activities. Fortunately, as we've seen countless times among the cadets at the United States Military Academy, good posture is not very difficult to achieve.

Standing: Good posture (while standing) involves holding your head high while simultaneously tucking in your chin. This action flattens the curve in your cervical spine. You should also pull your stomach in, roll your hips slightly backward (thereby tilting your pelvis slightly backward) and tighten your buttock muscles somewhat by contracting (squeezing) them (Figure 6–2). This maneuver flattens the curve in your

Figure 6–2   Achieving good posture

° Hold your head high. Tuck your chin in slightly. Stand tall.

° Relax your shoulders. Elevate your chest slightly. Hold your abdomen in. Your beltline should be horizontal to the ground.

° Bring your hips back over your ankles. Tuck your pelvis (tailbone) down.

° Keep your knees straight but not locked.

° Rock forward and back. Place your weight on your feet in the area in front of your ankle bone.

lumbar spine. Remember that good posture begins with your head and your pelvis — get them properly aligned and the rest of your body will fall into line. If you must stand for an extended period of time, don't stand in the same position for too long. You should periodically shift your weight and change positions. You should also support one foot above the other on a low stool or box, alternating your feet every so often (Figure 6-3).

Sitting: A proper sitting position is important — both at work and during periods of relaxation. The best basic position is one in which you keep your knees level with your hips and your feet flat on the floor. Your back should be firmly supported by the back of your chair. This support enables you to maintain the lordotic curve in your lower back without undue muscular effort on your part. The support can be provided by an external device (e.g., a small pillow or a rolled-up towel) or by an orthopedically designed chair (e.g., one with

Figure 6-3 If you must stand for an extended period of time, don't stand in the same position for too long.

lumbar back support built into it). If possible, the chair in which you choose to sit should have armrests, because the support provided by armrests helps to ease the load on your spine. Your chair should be adjustable in height so that you can attain the proper sitting position (especially if you have a job in which you sit most of the day). You should get up from your chair for five minutes at least once every half hour and move around. You should avoid slouching down in your chair. Although a slouched position may seem comfortable, it actually places additional stress on your back. You should also avoid leaning forward while sitting to work at a desk or table.

Sleeping: Since most of us spend approximately one-third of our lives in bed, it is little wonder that much has been written about choosing a mattress. To make the decision "easier" for you, manufacturers of mattresses frequently attach adjectives such as "orthopedic," "chiropractic" and "posture" to their products. The inference is obvious. Reportedly, these products — described in "medical" terms — have been scientifically designed and tested for anyone who cares to provide the best care for their back. The truth of the situation is another matter.

In the first place, there are no hard-and-fast rules with regard to the selection of a mattress. As simple as it sounds, what is best is whatever works best for you. Since most individuals suffering from back pain find a soft (sagging) bed to be uncomfortable, the traditional rule of thumb is that a relatively firm mattress is recommended for back pain sufferers. Some people, however, prefer a mattress that is less firm or even soft. You should test a variety of mattresses until you find one that is comfortable for *your* back.

In addition to selecting a mattress that is appropriate to your needs, you also should find a comfortable sleeping position. If you try a position and it isn't comfortable, try another. As a general rule, if you suffer from back pain, you should avoid sleeping on your stomach, since this position tends to exaggerate the curve in your lower back, thereby placing an unnecessary strain on your back. If you tend to sleep on your back, we recommend that you place a pillow under your knees. If you sleep on your side, you should bend you knees. If you are currently suffering from back pain, you should use as many pillows as necessary to keep your spine level while you sleep. A sagging spine can exacerbate the pain in your back. Your shoulders and hips should be in a vertical line.

If you're in pain, you should also decide what is the best way to get into and out of bed. The general rule of thumb is to do both movements slowly and gradually. Pain has a very sharp way of letting you know if you move too suddenly or too unknowingly. To get into bed, first sit on the side of the bed with your palms resting on the mattress. Then slowly lower your body sideways and simultaneously raise your legs so you end up lying on your side. Use your hands and then your forearms to ease your movements from sitting to lying, making every effort to avoid putting stress on your back. Once you are on your side, slowly move into your favorite position for sleeping. Getting out of bed simply involves doing the movements for getting into bed in reverse order. You should avoid twisting or bending your back while getting into or out of bed.

Walking: Good posture while walking involves the same basic elements of correct posture that standing does. Stand tall. Hold your head high. Keep your chin tucked in slightly. Pull your stomach in. Roll you hips slightly backward. Tighten you buttock muscles. If you carry a shoulder bag as you walk, switch the bag from shoulder to shoulder periodically.

Lifting: Many back injuries are caused by improper lifting techniques. As a general rule, you can avoid these injuries by being aware of and adhering to the 12 basic *rules of lifting.*

1. Stand close to the object you're lifting with your feet apart to ensure that you have firm footing.

2. Bend your knees. Keep your back as straight as possible by minimizing any bending at your waist. Bending at the waist increases the stress on your back.

3. Tighten your stomach muscles before you lift. Your abdominal muscles, as we mentioned in Chapter 1, can be considered as your anterior back muscles. They help to support your back.

3. Tighten your stomach muscles before you lift. Your abdominal muscles, as we mentioned in Chapter 1, can be considered as your anterior back muscles. They help to support your back.

4. Lift with your legs by slowly straightening them. Make your legs (not your back muscles) do the work.

5. Hold the (lifted) load close to your body. The farther away an object is held from your body, the greater the stress it will place on your back.

6. Keep your back in an upright position during the lift and while holding the object.

7. Reverse steps 1 through 6 to lower your load.

8. Avoid twisting your body while lifting. Move your feet if it's necessary to change directions or to see something not otherwise in view.

9. While carrying an object, move smoothly. Don't move suddenly or jerk your body.

10. Decide where you're going to go with the object you're going to lift before you lift it. Make sure that you have a clear path to reach that point before you lift the object.

11. Check the object to be lifted carefully for any possible impediments (e.g., a sharp or jagged edge) before you lift the object.

12. Get assistance when the object to be lifted is too heavy or too large.

Traveling: Guidelines for maintaining proper body mechanics while traveling depend on your mode of travel. If you're driving a car, we recommend that you push your car seat into a comfortable position as far forward as possible, so you can avoid over-reaching for the pedals. Whether you're the driver or a passenger in a car, you might consider putting a pillow or a rolled-up towel behind your back to support it. If your car seats are very soft and you prefer a more rigid seat, you should consider purchasing some type of device that will provide that rigidity. These devices vary widely in both cost and complexity. If you have to be in the car for an extended period of time, you should stop every hour or so and get out to stretch and walk around.

If you're traveling by plane, there are several options to consider in order to maintain a good position for your back. Like auto travel, you can place one or more small pillows (readily available on most commercial flights) behind your lower back to provide support. If you are short, you may find it necessary to take a carry-on piece of luggage to be used to prop up your feet once the flight is airborne. If you are tall, you should make every effort to get an aisle seat so that you can stretch your legs occasionally. You should also ask the reservations/seat assignment person if it would be possible to assign you a seat with extra leg room. On commercial flights, such seats are often adjacent to emergency exits and are called bulkhead seats. But whatever your height, you should periodically get up and walk around during the flight.

Sports

In the environment in which we work at West Point, almost everyone — cadets, staff and faculty and dependents — is an athlete of some sort. Ranging from the intercollegiate competitive sports teams of the cadets to the recreational noontime joggers, the vast majority of the West Point community engages in some level of regular physical activity. While the degree of enthusiasm for athletics or personal conditioning may not be quite as extensive or intense in your community, it would not be surprising if the majority of people you know like to work out or participate in sports.

Individuals who fall into the aforementioned category face several basic questions regarding the possible effects that physical exertion has on the health of their backs. What is the possible danger to your back from participating in a specific sport or conditioning activity? Is there anything that you can or should do to protect your back while participating? Is there anything that you can do *before* participating that will subsequently help your back?

Listing all the possible sports and conditioning activities in which you could engage would be a substantial undertaking. Developing a checklist of possible beneficial guidelines to protect your back while participating in those activities would be an even more extensive task. Identifying what you can do before you become an active participant is somewhat easier. Unquestionably, the most valuable action you can take is to get into as good a condition as possible (Figure 6–4). With regard to your back, this involves strengthening your abdominal muscles using a variety of the numerous exercises designed for conditioning your stomach muscles and strengthening your lower back muscles using the BackMate program. Healthy muscles are not only strong, but flexible. Maintaining your flexibility should also be an important aspect of your conditioning program. *Note:* There are over 30 separate

Figure 6–4   Properly conditioning and strengthening your lower back and abdominal muscles can help you avoid sports-related back pain.

calisthenic-type exercises for strengthening the stomach muscles. The sit-up is probably the most common one, but there are others that are more effective.

We also highly recommend that both before and while you are participating in sports and conditioning activities, you exercise a lot of common sense regarding your back. Be sure you have stretched and warmed up before exercising. Don't take any unreasonable chances. Table 6–1 illustrates the relative risks of incurring a back injury from participating in selected sports and fitness activities.

The question arises: What is reasonable? Obviously, "reasonable" is a relative term. What may be reasonable to us may be unreasonable to you. It's your back, your life and your decision. We do suggest, however, that you "listen" to your back. If it hurts, your back is sending you a message. Don't ignore it. You may need to make some changes in what you're doing. Probably the most sensible advice we could give you is that when deciding whether or not to participate in a specific activity, you should consider the pleasure-pain ratio—a subjectively quantitative measure first suggested by Dr. Augustus White in his best-selling book, *Your Aching Back*. White recommended that if the pleasure you derive from a sport exceeds the back pain you incur, then have at it. Within the limits of common sense, we agree.

Sexual Activity

In sexual relations, as in every other form of physical activity, the principles of sensible back care hold true. You and your partner must be aware of and use proper body mechanics while making love so as not to irritate your back. As you may well know, when your back pain is severe enough, movements associated with usual sexual activity may become almost impossible. Even when your back pain is not that severe, your fear that sexual activity may make your pain worse can inhibit you emotionally. For the record, there is no cause or factor related to back pain that is adversely affected by sexual activity. You need not fear that sex may, somehow, inflict permanent damage to your back.

Having learned that your risk of physiological harm from sexual activity is very unlikely, you should also be aware that, for some people, back pain has been known to cause either sexual dysfunction or make a preexisting sexual problem worse. There are isolated cases in which men have become impotent and women frigid because of back pain. There are also instances in which back pain has aggravated a preexisting state of emotional strain and hostility between individuals. In such cases a loss of sex drive may result. In all of these examples, the problems are essentially psychologically (emotionally) rooted.

What you and your partner need in these instances is a proper mixture of clear, honest communication; trust; patience and sympathetic understanding. Individuals who haven't been able to achieve that mix are advised to seek professional assistance.

There are several guidelines that you should consider if you or your partner has a back problem and you want to maintain a mutually satisfying sex life. For discussion purposes, these guidelines are grouped into two categories: consciousness and mechanical.

Table 6–1 The relative risks of incurring a back injury from participating in selected sports and fitness activities*

HIGH RISK ACTIVITIES	FOOTBALL GYMNASTICS POWER LIFTING WRESTLING
MEDIUM TO HIGH RISK ACTIVITIES	HANDBALL HOCKEY LACROSSE RACQUETBALL SQUASH

MEDIUM RISK ACTIVITIES	BASEBALL
	DANCE
	DIVING
	ROWING
	SOCCER
	TRACK & FIELD
	   – THROWING EVENTS
	   – RUNNING

LOW TO MEDIUM RISK ACTIVITIES	BASKETBALL BOXING DOWNHILL SKIING GOLF JOGGING STRENGTH TRAINING TENNIS VOLLEYBALL
LOW RISK ACTIVITIES	CROSS COUNTRY SKIING CYCLING HIKING SAILING SCUBA DIVING SWIMMING WALKING

*Note: You should keep in mind that there is a difference between relatively minor back pain that is muscle-related and a back injury. Participation in many of these sports and fitness activities can result in back pain; most, however, are not high risk in terms of their potential for causing a back injury.

Consciousness Guidelines

1. Start with a positive attitude. Your back pain is *not* going to keep you and your partner from having a satisfying sex life.

2. Talk to your partner. There simply is no substitute for honest, caring communication. Be as subtle or as frank as you'd like, but open the lines of direct communication as soon as possible.

3. Approach the problem of how to deal with your back pain, while maintaining a satisfying sex life, with a cooperative attitude. You and your partner must make a firm commitment to give and take, when necessary, to achieve the most satisfying experience for *both* of you. This will require a maximum degree of sympathetic understanding of what is pleasureable and what is painful for the other partner.

4. Be more open-minded about lovemaking. Expand your attitudes. Talk more. Touch more. Care more. Be more sensual. Lovemaking can, and should, involve more than coital activities.

5. Enjoy what you're doing while lovemaking if it doesn't hurt. If it does hurt, make a commitment to knowing and adhering to the following mechanical guidelines for making love when you have a back problem.

Mechanical Guidelines

1. Don't bend forward at the waist with your knees *straight* during sexual intercourse. Even if you're lying down, this position puts tremendous stress on your lower back. If you bend your knees, you can bend slightly forward.

2. Arch your lower back as little as possible, because arching your back places considerable force on the posterior structures of your spine.

3. Don't lie flat on your stomach or your back with your hips extended straight. This position over-stresses the hip flexor muscles that extend from the front of your lumbar spine to just below your hip joint. If these muscles are tense or taut, pressure is put on your lower back. You can relax these muscles by bending at the hips; flex (bend) one or both of your hips. Assuming a hips-flexed position will help protect your lower back from irritation.

4. Consider using one of the positions for sexual intercourse shown in Figures 6–5 to 6–9. Each of these positions is particularly suited for partners, one of whom has back pain.

Figure 6–5 This is the traditional basic position when either partner suffers from back pain. It is possibly the best lovemaking position to use when either partner's back pain is in the acute stage.

Figure 6–6 This position is good when the woman suffers from back pain. The woman's upper torso should be supported with pillows and her thighs should be supported by her partner's arms and thighs.

Figure 6–7 This position is good when the woman suffers from back pain. This can also be a good position for a man with back pain, provided his upper torso is raised slightly (with pillows) in order to flex his spine.

Figure 6–8

This position is good when the man suffers from back pain. Note that his back is slightly flexed, as opposed to extended. This is not a good position for a woman with back pain.

Figure 6–9

This position is good when the man suffers from back pain. This is not a good position when the woman has back pain.

Once you understand and make a reasonable attempt to adhere to the aforementioned guidelines, is there anything else you can do? Keeping in mind that this text is not intended to be a lovemaking manual and that we are not particularly qualified to write one, we offer the following additional suggestions for you to consider. If you have back pain, your partner should be the one to provide any motion during sexual intercourse. If your pain is greater than your pleasure during lovemaking, then you or your partner must make an appropriate adaptation in either body position or technique. When you irritate your back, pain is your body's way of keeping you informed that you're doing something that is over-stressing your back. And finally, in view of the wide array of pleasureable alternatives for achieving a satisfying sex life, even for those individuals with back pain, the old adage "where there's a will there's a way" may apply.

MAINTAINING BODY LEANNESS

If by shedding extra pounds you reduce the load that your spine must carry around and your back muscles must support, you reduce the stress your back must handle. At the same time, you decrease the likelihood that you will suffer from back pain. Keeping your weight at an appropriate level can also have a positive effect on your posture. A protruding stomach frequently leads to lordosis (swayback), a condition that places considerable stress on the posterior elements of the spine. A flat, muscularly fit stomach, on the other hand, lends itself to the maintenance of proper body mechanics. As we mentioned earlier, your stomach muscles play an important role in supporting your back. For that reason, they are frequently referred to as your "anterior back muscles."

Before offering suggestions on how you might approach the process of shedding excess poundage, we'd like to

Figure 6–10   Measuring a person's body fat with a pair of calipers

explain the difference between two very important terms: overweight and overfat. It is important that you understand the precise meanings of these terms if you are to maintain body leanness. Being *overweight* simply means weighing more than other individuals of the same height and age. Being *overfat,* on the other hand, means you have more body fat than you should for your good health. Overfat is an indication of poor fitness. Overweight, on the other hand, is not an accurate indicator of fitness because some people simply have more muscle (and bone) than the average person.

An excellent example of this is the muscularly-developed professional athlete who would be considered overweight but not overfat.

Unfortunately, many individuals are concerned only with how much they weigh rather than how much body fat they have. For your health and fitness, it is not how much you weigh that is important, but how much of your body is lean muscle and bone and how much is fat (adipose tissue). The component of fitness that relates to what percentage of your body weight is fat and what percentage is muscle mass and bone is commonly referred to as *body leanness*. At West Point, the maximum allowable percent of body fat for men and women cadets is 18 percent and 26 percent respectively. For society in general, the upper range of percent body fat is, regrettably, much higher. All individuals would be healthier and would have backs much less likely to suffer the rigors of pain if they maintained a proper level of body leanness. In some instances, individuals develop extremely high levels of body fat. Once men and women reach body fat levels of 30 percent and 35 percent respectively, they are considered to be *obese*. Obesity is a sure ticket on a train ride to poor health. It should be avoided without exception.

How to Lose Body Fat

No magic formula exists for fat loss. The *only* sound method for losing fat is to expend more calories or energy than you consume. As a process, maintaining body leanness can be viewed as the end product of two antagonistic forces on a scale (Table 6–2):

ENERGY IN   **ENERGY OUT**

Energy In = Calories received from various foods eaten. These amounts vary according to their fat, carbohydrate and protein content.

Energy Out = The energy the body uses to exist. The amount of energy used for various functions is generally dependent upon the amount of the body's large musculature that is involved in the activity. The greater the involvement, the larger the energy cost; e.g., an individual burns approximately 30 calories per hour while sleeping and 900 calories per hour while running (at 10 mph).

- If energy in is greater than energy out, you will *increase* body fat.
- If energy out is greater than energy in, you will *decrease* body fat.
- If energy out is equal to energy in, you will experience *no change* in body fat.

Table 6–2 The relationship between energy in and energy out

Since a pound of body fat contains approximately 3,500 calories, if you want to lose two pounds per week, the energy in must be 7,000 *fewer* calories than the energy out. This negative balance can be achieved in one of three ways: 1) by burning up an additional 7,000 calories per week (via exercise), 2) by cutting back 7,000 calories on your total weekly caloric intake (dieting), or 3) through a combination of both exercising and dieting. The latter alternative is the most feasible because it does not involve an unreasonable expenditure of either time or self-discipline on your part. Remember that the key to weight control is *moderation.* Do not starve yourself. You didn't raise your percentage of body fat to an unacceptable level overnight, and you won't lower it overnight. Become familiar with caloric values of the foods that are accessible to you. Calorie charts are sold at the checkout counters of most grocery stores. Learn the caloric expenditure totals for the various physical activities in which you might participate. Table 6–3 lists the approximate calorie expenditure by individuals of different body weights in selected physical activities. Calculate your approximate total weekly caloric intake. Next, develop a plan for a proper diet and exercise to achieve a one- to two-pound weight loss per week. Remember, maintaining body leanness is *your* responsibility. Once you attain an acceptable body fat level, you should continue to exercise and eat wisely in order to preserve what you have achieved. You owe it to your back to make a commitment to good health.

General Suggestions for Losing Body Fat

The number of books in print dealing with how to lose "weight" is only exceeded by books on religion and cookbooks. Most of the diet books tend to offer the reader a relatively painless approach for losing fat. Claims, counterclaims, gimmicks and the like notwithstanding, all sensible weight (fat) control efforts can be summarized in just five words: *EAT LESS AND EXERCISE MORE.* No magic formula. No quick and easy techniques. Just plain old common sense and the willpower to adhere to basic nutritional guidelines. Although any listing of the possible actions you could take to help maintain your body leanness at an acceptable level would be almost endless, we suggest that you consider the following steps for losing body fat.

1. Exercise regularly and vigorously. Exercises and activities involving much of the body's large musculature and lasting for extended periods of time are recommended. If your back pain presently limits the amount of time you feel like exercising, your BackMate program will help you get more involved in exercising on a routine basis.

2. Moderation is the key to weight control. Be aware of how much you eat and take sensible steps to eat moderate amounts of food.

3. Eat a balanced diet. Be sure that you get enough of the essential nutrients for good health. The U.S. Department of Agriculture recommends that everyone have a daily serving from the "Basic Four" to assure a balanced diet: 1) meat, fish, poultry and eggs; 2) milk and milk products; 3) vegetables and fruits; 4) bread and cereals.

4. Decrease your caloric intake. If you cut back 100 calories a day (e.g., a single slice of bread) less than your needs, you will lose 10–12 pounds per year.

5. Learn to eat slowly in order to learn to eat less. Put your fork or spoon down on the table between bites of food. Chew your food thoroughly.

6. Limit the portions of food you eat at meals to one average (reasonable) serving.

7. Omit or restrict free fats such as butter, margarine, mayonnaise, and ice cream.

8. Omit or restrict free sweets such as pastries and candy.

9. Eat regular meals. Your total caloric intake affects your weight, but the number of meals you eat per day does *not*. Do not eliminate breakfast. Physiologically, breakfast is the most important meal of the day. If you want to reduce your caloric intake by cutting down on the size of your meals, reduce your food intake at lunch or dinner.

10. Avoid "empty calories," expecially after the dinner meal. Alcohol is a particularly useless and unneeded source of calories.

11. Weigh yourself daily and keep a written record of your weight. Use the same scale each time and weigh yourself at approximately the same time each day.

12. Eliminate foods needlessly high in calories (e.g., cut the fat off of steak, abstain from putting sugar in your coffee or tea, abstain from using sour cream on your potatoes, limit your intake of alcoholic beverages, abstain from using gravy).

13. Minimize all snacking between meals. If you must eat something between meals, try to eat a sensible snack like raw vegetables or fruit.

14. Avoid diets which concentrate on a single nutrient or which omit certain nutrients altogether. Both types of diets are very dangerous, don't work in the long run and should be avoided at all costs.

15. Do not severely limit your caloric intake. Diets in which you ingest fewer than 1,000 calories per day should only be undertaken with the supervision of a physician. Long-term fasting is particularly detrimental to your health.

EXERCISE

Muscles and ligaments are the common denominator of painful backs. As a result, the single most important therapeutic measure in the vast majority of instances of back pain is proper exercise. Unfortunately, it is somewhat difficult to convince back pain victims of that fact and to get them to engage in a regular program of exercise.

Table 6–3 Caloric expenditure in various activities

ACTIVITY	CALORIES BURNED PER HOUR		
	BODY WEIGHT		
	100 LBS	150 LBS	200 LBS
ARCHERY	180	240	300
BACKPACKING (40 LB PACK)	305	410	515
BADMINTON	255	340	425
BASEBALL	210	280	350
BASKETBALL (HALF COURT)	225	300	375
BICYCLING (10 MPH)	300	480	600
BOWLING	155	210	260
CANOEING (4 MPH)	275	415	560
DANCE, AEROBIC	355	540	625
DANCE, SOCIAL	210	280	350
FENCING	225	300	375
FITNESS CALISTHENICS	235	310	390
FOOTBALL	225	300	375
GOLF (WALKING)	185	250	315
GYMNASTICS	230	310	390
HANDBALL	450	600	750
HIKING	225	300	375
JOGGING (5 1/2 MPH)	490	650	835
MARTIAL ARTS	230	310	390
MOUNTAIN CLIMBING	450	600	750
RACQUETBALL	450	600	750
ROPE JUMPING (CONTINUOUS)	525	700	875
ROWING	615	820	1025
RUNNING	625	900	1125
SAILING	135	180	225
SKATING, ICE	265	350	440
SKATING, ROLLER	265	350	440
SKIING, CROSS COUNTRY	525	700	875
SKIING, DOWNHILL	450	600	750
SOCCER	405	540	575
SOFTBALL (FAST)	210	280	350
SOFTBALL (SLOW)	220	290	370
STRENGTH TRAINING	350	470	560
SWIMMING (FAST LAPS)	420	630	850
SWIMMING (SLOW LAPS)	240	320	400
TABLE TENNIS	180	240	300
TENNIS	315	420	525
VOLLEYBALL	260	350	485
WALKING	160	210	265
WATERSKIING	360	480	600

Figure 6–11 Exercise is beneficial for muscles and ligaments.

To fully comprehend the importance of exercise in treating and preventing back pain, you need to understand that much of the strength of your spine does not come from the bones of your spine. On the contrary, the muscles of your spine and the strapping effect of the spine's ligaments provide the foundation of strength for your spine. Muscles and ligaments are affected in a positive way by exercise. Of particular importance is the fact that exercise increases the strength and efficiency of your lower back muscles. Exercise also strengthens and firms your abdominal muscles, thereby reducing the level of stress on the posterior structures of your back caused by a weak or protruding stomach. Finally, some exercises are designed to stretch your lower back and leg muscles. By eliminating the tightness in your muscles, stretching exercises often relieve much of the stress with which your back must deal. Flexible, relaxed muscles are better able to handle the demands for dynamic movements that are frequently placed upon them.

What Exercises Should You Do?

The literature is replete with suggestions on what exercises you should do to treat and prevent back pain. There are almost as many theories as there are different people willing to espouse an opinion on what you should do. In our opinion, any sensible exercise program for back pain will include both stretching and strengthening exercises. Your strengthening regimen should include exercises for both your abdominal region and your lower back. Identifying which exercises to do is largely a matter of personal preference. Whatever exercises you select, however, they should be relatively simple to do and should not place any undue stress on your back.

At West Point, we recommend doing the BackMate program to strengthen the extensor muscles of your lower back and the six exercises illustrated in Figures 6–13 through 6–18 to develop the flexor muscles of your lower back. Of the two muscle groups, the extensors appear to play a much more critical role in the treatment and prevention of back pain. Before our efforts with the BackMate when this approach to treating back pain was discovered, there was an almost complete lack of safe, effective exercises for developing the extensor muscles of the lower back. Since no one was able to determine how to develop the extensor muscles of the lower back, these muscles have been virtually ignored in most therapeutic exercise programs.

Figures 6–19 through 6–24 illustrate six stretching exercises, and Figures 6–25 through 6–30 illustrate six abdominal exercises. Keep in mind that the number of possible stretching and strengthening exercises is great. The exercises included in these tables represent those which we have found to work well for individuals with back pain.

Figure 6–12   A regular exercise program can benefit people of all ages.

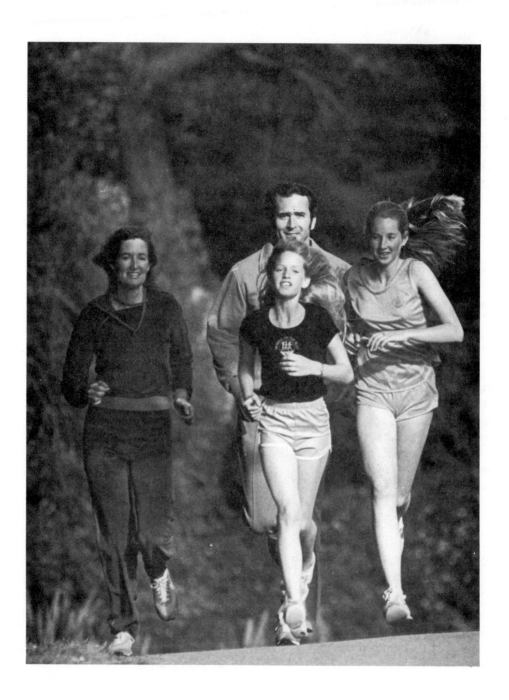

Figures 6–13 through 6–18   Exercises to develop the flexor muscles of the lower back

Figure 6–13 Pelvic Tilt

Tighten your stomach and roll the top of your pelvis backward. You should feel the small of your back flatten. Hold for 15 seconds. Practice holding your back flat while sitting, standing and walking.

Figure 6–14   Single Knee to Shoulder

Grasp behind your right knee and slowly pull your knee toward your right shoulder. You should feel a gentle stretch on the right side of your back. Hold for 15 seconds. Breathe normally. Alternate with your left knee to your left shoulder.

Figure 6–15 Double Knee to Shoulder

Grasp behind both knees; slowly pull them toward your shoulders. You should feel a gentle stretch in the small of your back. Hold for 15 seconds. Breathe normally.

Figure 6–16   Partial Sit -up

Do a pelvic tilt and hold it. Tuck your chin and curl forward until your shoulder blades just leave the floor. You should feel your stomach muscles working. Hold for five seconds. Breathe normally. Slowly lower yourself back to the floor.

Figure 6–17   Hip Flexor Stretch

Do a pelvic tilt and hold it. Grasp behind your right knee and pull it toward your right shoulder. Flatten your left thigh against the floor. You should feel your left buttock tighten and a stretch at the top front of your thigh. Hold for 15 seconds. Breathe normally. Alternate sides.

Figure 6–18   Flexion Resting Posture

Lie on your back with your calves resting on a chair seat. Completely relax. You should feel the small of your back flatten. Remain in this position for 15 seconds.

Figures 6–19 through 6–24   Sample stretching exercises

Figure 6–19

Sit down with your heels 8 to 10 inches apart. With your legs straight, slowly bend forward at your waist. Hold an easy stretch for 10 seconds. Then slightly increase your stretch by bending forward even more. Hold for another 10 seconds.

Figure 6–20

From a standing position, place one leg in front of the other. Keeping both of your legs straight, bend at your waist slowly. Repeat and alternate legs.

Figure 6–21

From a sitting position, place one ankle on the knee of your opposite leg. Try to touch your chest to the knee of your straight leg; hold and alternate legs.

Figure 6–22   Sit with your legs stretched out as far as possible without straining. Keep your feet upright and relaxed. Now slowly lean straight forward until you feel a strain on the inside of your legs. Next, stretch your hamstring and back muscles by bending your waist toward your foot. Keep your head up. Hold for 10 seconds; alternate legs.

Figure 6–23

Pull the soles of your feet together. With your hands clasped around your feet, slowly pull yourself forward until you feel a stretch in your groin area. Hold an easy stretch for 10 seconds. Slowly increase the stretch as you feel yourself relax. Keep your elbows on the outside of your legs for greater stability.

Figure 6–24

Sit on the floor or on a stool with your back straight. Clasp your hands behind your neck. Have a partner stand behind you. Twist your trunk as far as possible while you look over your right shoulder. Have your partner push on your left shoulder and pull gently backward on your right elbow. Hold the position for 10 seconds. Alternate to the other side.

Figures 6–25 through 6–30   Sample exercises to develop the abdominal muscles

Figure 6–25

Stand with your feet shoulder width apart, your arms extended up over your head and your hands clasped together. Keep your arms close to your head and slowly bend to the side, pause, return to the center, and bend to the other side. Repeat right, center, left, center, right, etc. Note: keep your hips stable.

Figure 6–26

On your hands and knees with your back straight, tuck your chin to your chest and raise your back up as you pull in your stomach muscles (arch your back like a cat when it stretches). Relax and repeat. Note: do not let your back sag at any time during the exercise.

Figure 6–27

From a back-lying position, do a pelvic tilt. Then straighten out your left leg and press it flat to the floor while keeping your knee rigid. Then without using your hands and arms for leverage, raise your straightened leg as high as you can until you can feel a tightness in your thigh. After your leg is as high as you can comfortably raise it, hold for a count of five. Then, while you keep your knee straight, slowly let your leg return to the floor. Relax, then repeat with the other leg. Alternate legs for 10 repetitions.

Figure 6–28

Assume a back-lying position with your knees bent and your feet flat on the floor. Your hands may rest on your shoulders or your fingers may be interlocked behind your back. Slowly curl your head toward your knees and continue curling up until your elbows touch your knees.

Figure 6–29

Assume a back-lying position with your arms held out at your shoulders. Slowly raise your left leg up (toes pointed) and lower it across your body toward your right hand. If this is too difficult, touch the floor at your waist level or above. Slowly return your leg to a straight-up position and lower it to the floor. Repeat with your right leg, left, right, etc. Note: Keep your back, head, and shoulders in contact with the floor as much as possible during the exercise.

Figure 6–30

Sit with your legs together, toes pointed and hands on your shoulders. Twist your trunk to the right, and continue twisting for four counts while you look over your right shoulder. Repeat to your left, right, left, etc. Note: Do not let your hips turn while you do the exercise. You are in a seated rather than a standing position to stabilize your hips so they cannot assist with the twisting action of your trunk.

How Should You Organize Your Exercise Program?

Although there are no set ways of organizing an exercise program for treating and preventing back pain, several guidelines exist to help you increase the levels of safety, efficiency and effectiveness of your therapeutic exercise program.

Before beginning your exercise program, you should consult a physician to make sure that the exercises won't aggravate your condition. This caution is particularly important if you are experiencing severe pain. Unlike traditional advice on when to begin your exercise program, we recommend doing BackMate exercises as soon as it is determined that the basic cause of your pain is not a fracture, an infection or a tumor. We have had people who are in the midst of excruciating back pain work out on BackMate and experience immediate relief, ranging from partial to total. To date, we have not had a single instance in which the BackMate exercises aggravated an individual's back pain, even one suffering from muscle spasms or sciatica. On the other hand, if doing the exercises—including BackMate—increases your pain, you should consult your physician before continuing with your exercise program. There may be something seriously wrong with your back which previously was undetected.

The schedule of when and how long to do each exercise varies somewhat from individual to individual. Common sense dictates that you should stretch before and after doing the strengthening exercises. If you're doing the BackMate program, the prescribed BackMate protocol is designed to provide both before and after stretching. If, on the other hand, you're doing traditional calisthenic-type stretching and strengthening exercises, you'll need to establish an appropriate order for doing the exercises. The number of repetitions and sets you should perform of each exercise, how many times a day you should exercise and how many times a week you should work out also vary according to your personal perspective of "how much exercise is too much." At West Point, the general philosophy is that *more (exercise) is not necessarily better.*

We recommend performing a single set of 10–12 repetitions of each exercise, three times a week (on alternative days)—unless you're currently suffering from back pain. In that instance, you may need or want to work out every day. We actually have had individuals who worked out on BackMate several times a day because exercising on BackMate provided the only relief that they could obtain while still attempting to lead a normal life. Whatever the "number recipe" you finally decide is best for your needs, remember that exercise is not a contest. Don't focus on how much you lift or how many repetitions you can do. Just do the program in the proper fashion. If you exercise properly, there are no losers.

BACK PROBLEMS PARTICULAR TO WOMEN

There are some problems relating to back pain that only women have. A noninclusive list of these problems includes menstruation, pregnancy and postnatal back.

Menstruation

In some instances, just before a woman's menstrual period begins, her uterus puts extra pressure on her back because the uterine walls become heavier with the buildup of the lining of the walls. As a result, menstrual periods almost always make a low back condition worse. In addition, most women tend to retain extra fluids throughout their body during the time of their menstrual period. The extra fluids often cause a weight gain of three to ten pounds. More often than not, the extra weight is carried in the stomach. This extra weight produces even more stress on the lower back.

If you experience an increase in low back pain or a substantial weight gain during your menstrual period, we recommend that you eat a high protein diet for approximately ten days, commencing five days before the start of your period. A diet high in protein tends to lessen fluid retention. To minimize the level of stress placed on your lower back by your heavier-than-normal stomach, it is important that you develop very strong abdominal muscles. There is additional nutritional evidence that your diet at this time should also include foodstuffs high in iron and roughage. Nutritionists suggest that such a diet should help give you better control over you abdominal muscles.

One final note on this subject involves the use of tampons. Although the use of tampons causes no trouble for most women, some women cannot use tampons of any kind because they cause back pain. If you're experiencing back pain during your menstrual period, you should consider switching to sanitary napkins. Each individual's level of sensitivity to intrauterine devices (e.g., tampons, diaphragms, IUDs) is different. If you're suffering from low back pain during your menstrual period, you should check out every possibility.

Pregnancy

Pregnancy more often than not causes back pain in expectant mothers as they approach the end of their term. This pain is essentially the result of the mechanical forward adjustment of a pregnant woman's spine which occurs as her increased size shifts her center of gravity forward. As a result, her lower back is forced to deal with greater than normal stresses. In addition, a pregnant woman also must confront the problems caused by mechanical changes in her sacroiliac and other joints. These changes are produced by her body's release of a hormone called relaxin. Relaxin loosens the pelvic ligaments as a precursor to permitting her baby's head to move more easily through her pelvic canal during birth. Like all adjustments to proper body mechanics, these changes place further stress on the pregnant woman's lower back. Coupled with the gradual lessening of her control over her abdominal muscles (the anterior muscles of the back), it is little wonder that back pain is prevalent among expectant mothers.

The program to prevent or at least minimize back pain for expectant mothers is threefold. First, a pregnant woman should strengthen her lower back and abdominal muscles as much as possible. Before commencing her exercise program, an expectant mother should consult her physician to determine an exercise regimen to follow.

Second, an expectant mother should be particularly sensitive to proper body mechanics and adhere to them at all times. Finally, an expectant mother should include extra periods of rest (lying down) in her schedule in order to reduce the cumulative amount of stress in her lower back.

Postnatal Back

Right after a woman has given birth, her pelvic ligaments are loosened, the strength of her abdominal muscles is normally quite low and her lower back muscles are usually both tightened and fatigued from the previous months of dealing with the extra stress that was placed upon them. Along with the immediate need to perform the physical demands of carrying, lifting and lowering a new addition to her family, the lowered physical state of a woman in the postnatal period can have catastrophic effects on her back. The solution is similar to the proposed recommendations for dealing with the low back demands of pregnancy. In order to keep the degeneration of her physical state during pregnancy to a minimum, a woman should engage in a sensible exercise program prior to giving birth and for as long a period of time as her physician feels is appropriate for her. Once she gives birth, a woman should recommence her exercise program as soon as possible. Unless there were medical complications during delivery (e.g., caesarean section, hemorrhaging), the time to start an exercise program is *now*. Because the individual doing the exercise is responsible for exerting the force (at her own pace), the BackMate program is particularly well-suited for women undertaking a postnatal exercise program. Finally, in order to be able to minimize the physical demands imposed on her back by handling her baby, a woman needs to be aware of and adhere to proper body mechanics at all times. She should learn how to lift, lower and carry her baby in the manner that is least stressful to her back.

7

WHAT SHOULD YOU DO? QUESTIONS AND ANSWERS RELATING TO BACK PAIN

"No question is ever settled until it is settled right."

–Ella Wheeler Wilcox

This chapter is devoted to answering some of the questions concerning back pain that we've encountered over the years. Since individuals with back pain tend to have similar problems, chances are that the information presented in this chapter will enlighten you on most of the points concerning back pain that may require further clarification.

Q: Is there such a thing as risk-free surgery?

A. No. Although in most spinal operations there is a very small risk that problems will develop, there is always some risk involved.

Q: Would you recommend fusion for back pain diagnosed as idiopathic in nature?

A: No. All too often, fusion either fails to relieve the symptoms for which it is performed, or it actually makes them worse. In general, we would recommend fusion only to correct documented instability present in the spine, such as may occur as the consequences of trauma or from certain congenital defects.

Q: What is the best sport for someone who has back pain?

A: Choose a sport that you enjoy doing and one in which the pleasure you derive from your participation exceeds any pain that may result. Obviously, you shouldn't engage in any sport that places undue stress on your back. For example, tobogganing and touch football shouldn't be on your weekend activity schedule if you have severe back pain.

Q: What are the primary clues for determining the cause of back pain?

A: The clues are: the location of your pain, the precipitating event that caused your pain, when your back hurts and what makes the pain in your back increase or decrease.

Q: Is acupuncture an effective treatment for back pain?

A: Acupuncture appears to work for some patients, some of the time. Until research provides a documented answer regarding its benefits and risks, we don't recommend it.

Q: What is the approximate incidence of psychosomatic back pain?

A: The number of individuals who have back pain of a nonorganic nature has been estimated to be as high as 40–50 percent of all those suffering from back pain. You should keep in mind that the pain suffered by someone with psychosomatic back pain is every bit as "real" as the pain suffered by someone with back pain caused by trauma.

Q: *What is the pelvic tilt?*

A: Essentially, the pelvic tilt is an exercise that involves a movement very similar to the pelvic motion basic to lovemaking. This exercise is designed to strengthen your anterior spine structure and to stretch the posterior spine structure.

Q: *Can an individual with chronic back pain ever be able to have a satisfying sex life?*

A: As you well know, a satisfactory sex life is no small achievement, even for someone with a pain-free back. If you have back pain, you are going to have to be aware of certain adjustments that you may have to make in your lovemaking techniques if you are to have a satisfying love life. Refer to Chapter 6 for a discussion of some of the factors that should be considered.

Q: *Can an apparatus as apparently simple as the BackMate really help someone in back pain?*

A: We often make an analogy between the BackMate and the Heimlich maneuver. The first time most people see the Heimlich maneuver, they tend to be surprised at how simple but effective it is. Furthermore, most people are amazed that something as basic and as successful as the Heimlich maneuver wasn't discovered much earlier. These same reactions could easily occur when you see the Backmate exercises and realize that the BackMate program has been extraordinarily effective in treating back pain.

Q: *Is it possible that an automobile accident can produce an injury to someone's back that won't manifest itself until months or years later?*

A: This almost never happens. If your pain or lower back condition didn't appear within 48 hours or so after the accident, chances are that the accident isn't the cause of your back pain.

Q: Should X-rays be taken whenever someone has back pain?

A: The use of X-rays for individuals with minor back problems should be minimal, if they are used at all. Some physicians use X-rays in these situations merely to reassure the patient. No practical information is provided by X-rays in cases of minor back pain. In more serious cases of back complaints, X-rays serve a useful function.

Q: What is a myelogram?

A: A myelogram is an X-ray taken after a clear, water-soluble solution (somewhat misnamed as a dye) is injected into the watery, fluid-containing sac surrounding the nerves of the spine. This solution obstructs the passage of X-rays and enables the spinal canal to be outlined in such a way as to reveal anything causing substantial pressure on the nerve roots.

Q: Do you recommend using aspirin when back pain initially strikes an individual?

A: Unless an individual is aspirin-sensitive, most definitely yes. Aspirin acts as both a painkiller and as an anti-inflammatory to reduce back pain. The recommended approach for an adult when back pain initially strikes is to take the maximum dose: three aspirin every four hours.

Q: Should a person with back pain use a waterbed?

A: Some backs like waterbeds, some don't. The only hard-and-fast rule is to use what works for you.

Q: What does the term "conservative treatment" mean?

A: Traditionally, this term means nonsurgical treatment. Frankly, we would like to think that *all* back therapy—surgical and nonsurgical alike—is based on a considered, somewhat cautious perspective.

Accordingly, nonsurgical treatment should be rightfully referred to as nonoperative or nonsurgical therapy.

Q: *How much of what is known about back pain applies to neck pain?*

A: Quite a bit. Anatomically speaking, your neck is simply an extension of your spine. Some neck problems, however, are different in both quality and kind from back problems.

Q: *Does a difference in the lengths of a person's legs cause back pain?*

A: Moderate differences — as much as three-fourths of an inch to an inch — have no effect on your back.

Q: *Who is more likely to suffer from a herniated disc, men or women?*

A: Men. Men, for whatever reason, are also more likely than women to undergo surgery for back conditions of equal severity.

Q: *What are natural painkillers?*

A: Our bodies produce their own painkillers, called endorphins. The natural version of morphine, endorphins are chemicals released by the brain to dull pain.

Q: *Does your mind play a role in treating back pain?*

A: Most definitely. Your mind and your body work together when it comes to pain. By cooperating consciously with your treatment and by believing in your mind's healing powers, you can have a significant effect on your back. Don't let a negative attitude devastate your life.

Q: Would BackMate help an older person?

A: Age is obviously relative. When we were teenagers, we all thought anyone over 30 was old. Once we're over 30, we know better. But, the answer to the question is yes, BackMate will help an "older" person to either treat or prevent back pain. As we get older, our muscles tend to become more inflexible. In general, they also tend to get weaker as we slow down the pace of our lives. The BackMate's stretching and strengthening exercises can help to combat both tendencies.

Q: What is the best position for lying in bed for someone with a sore back?

A: In general, you should lie either on your side with your hips and knees bent or on your back, again with your hips and knees bent. The one position that you should definitely avoid is lying on your stomach.

Q: What kind of heat should someone with back pain use to treat the pain?

A: As long as it isn't too hot and doesn't damage the skin, any form of heat is acceptable. An electric heating pad is as good as anything.

Q: What does heat do for someone with back pain?

A: No one is absolutely certain what heat does. What is certain is that heat helps to soothe your pain. In turn, the continuous cycle of muscle spasm causing pain, causing more muscle spasm, etc. is often broken by the application of heat. It is not known whether or not this change occurs because heat blocks the transmission of pain or because heat causes circulatory changes under the skin.

Q: When should an individual return to work after an acute bout of back pain?

A: Unfortunately, there is no set answer to this question. On one hand, you don't want to delay returning to your normal lifestyle any longer than is necessary. On the other hand, you don't want to aggravate or prolong your condition needlessly by returning to work too soon. Ultimately, your decision should be based on your doctor's advice and your own assessment of your back pain.

Q: *IS DMSO an effective agent for the treatment of back pain?*

A: DMSO is an acronym for dimethyl sulfoxide, a substance that has been used to treat animals (particularly horses) for many years. We don't recommend it, and its benefits have not been documented. Fortunately, its usage hit its peak in the late seventies and early eighties and appears to be on a dramatic downswing.

Q: *What are the chances that an individual who has suffered back pain previously will have another bout?*

A: The chances are very good. Statistically, the chances are 60–70 percent that you will have a second bout of back pain within two years of your initial bout. If you strengthen and stretch the muscles supporting the spine, your chances of suffering another bout will be greatly reduced. We have had great success in preventing subsequent problems with back pain by using the BackMate.

Q: *What is the best drug for back pain?*

A: The best drug is aspirin or buffered aspirin. Table 4–1 in Chapter 4 presents a listing of the various drugs used to treat back pain and he effect of these drugs.

Q: *Can vibrating chairs, beds or hand massages help relieve back pain?*

A: Massaging agents (chairs, beds or hand-held vibrators) can certainly soothe your back and relax tense muscles. Massage tends to have the same effects as the application of heat.

Q: What kind of doctor should someone with back pain see for treatment?

A: Initially, you should see your family doctor. Your doctor may then refer you to a specialist — an orthopedic surgeon, a neurosurgeon or a rheumatologist.

Q: What is traction?

A: As it relates to treating back pain, traction is a form of back therapy in which the upper and lower parts of your body are pulled in opposite directions in order to ease your back pain. There are a number of theories as to how traction actually reduces back pain. What is known is that for a number of people, traction provides relief, albeit temporary, from back pain.

BIBLIOGRAPHY

Anderson, B. J. "A Quantitative Study of Back Loads in Lifting." *Spine* 1 (1976): 178–85.

Basmajian, J. V. *Grant's Method of Anatomy.* 8th ed. Baltimore: Williams and Wilkins Company, 1975.

Becker, F. R., James Wilson and J. A. Gehweiler. *The Anatomical Basis of Medical Practice.* Baltimore: Williams and Wilkins Company, 1971.

Benson, Herbert. *The Relaxation Response.* New York: William Morrow and Company, 1975.

Burkholz, Herbert. "Pain: Solving the Mystery." *The New York Times Magazine* 27 September 1987: 16–19, 32–35.

Cailliet, Rene. *Low Back Pain Syndrome.* 2nd ed. Philadelphia: F. A. Davis Company, 1974.

Caldwell, A. B. and C. Chase. "Diagnosis and Treatment of Personality Factors in Chronic Low Back Pain." *Clinical Orthopedics* 129 (1977): 141–49.

Chaffin, D. B. "Human Strength Capacity and Low Back Pain." *Journal of Occupational Medicine* 16 (1974): 248.

Cousins, Norman. *Anatomy of an Illness as Perceived by the Patient.* New York: Bantam Books, 1981.

Finneson, Bernard E. *Low Back Pain.* Philadelphia: J. B. Lippincott Company, 1981.

Fordyce, W. E., et al. "Pain Management and Pain Behavior." *Pain* 18 (1984): 53–69.

Friedmann, Lawrence W. and Lawrence Galton. *Freedom From Backaches.* New York: Pocket Books, 1973.

Gracovetsky, S. and H. Fartan. "The Optimum Spine." *Spine* Number 6. 11 (1986): 543–73.

Harris, D. V. and B. L. Harris. *The Athlete's Guide to Sports Psychology.* Champaign, IL: Leisure Press, 1984.

Hoeger, Warner W. *Lifetime Physical Fitness and Wellness.* Englewood, CO: Morton Publishing Company, 1986.

Hytten, Frank E. and Isabella Leitch. *The Physiology of Human Pregnancy.* Oxford, England: Blackwell Scientific Publications, 1964.

Isselbacher, K. J., R. D. Adams, E. Braunwald, R. G. Petersdort and J. D. Wilson, eds. *Principles of Internal Medicine.* New York: McGraw-Hill Book Company, 1980.

Jayson, M. I. V. *The Lumbar Spine and Back Pain.* Tunbridge Wells, England: Pitman Medical Publisher, 1980.

Krusen, Frank H., ed. *Handbook of Physical Medicine and Rehabilitation.* 2nd. ed. Philadelphia: W. B. Saunders Company, 1971.

Lettvin, Maggie. *Maggie's Back Book.* Boston: Houghton Mifflin Company, 1976.

Licht, Sidney, ed. *Rehabilitation and Medicine.* Baltimore: Waverly Press, 1968.

Lonetto, Richard and Gayle Kumchy. *Back to Normal.* Toronto: Doubleday and Company, 1986.

Macnab, Ian. *Backache.* Baltimore: Williams and Wilkins Company, 1977.

Masters, W. H. and V. Johnson. *Human Sexual Inadequacy.* Boston: Little, Brown and Company, 1970.

Melzack, R. and P. D. Wall. "Pain Mechanisms: A New Theory." *Science* 150 (1965): 971–79.

Mountcastle, Vernon B. *Medical Physiology.* 14th ed. St. Louis, MO: C. V. Mosby Company, 1980.

Nachemson, A. L. "The Lumbar Spine—An Orthopaedic Challenge." *Spine* 1 (1976):59.

Norton, P. L. and T. Brown. "The Immobilizing Efficiency of Back Braces." *Journal of Bone Joint Surgery* 39A (1957): 111.

Osborne, D. and T. Maruta. "Sexual Adjustment and Chronic Back Pain." *Medical Aspects of Human Sexuality* 14 (1980): 104–13.

Pelletier, Kenneth R. *Mind as Healer, Mind as Slayer.* New York: DEU, 1977.

Peterson, James A. and Susan L. Peterson. *The Sexy Stomach.* West Point, NY: Leisure Press, 1983.

Root, Leon and Thomas Kiernan. *Oh, My Aching Back.* New York: New American Library, 1985.

Sarno, John. *Mind Over Back Pain.* New York: Berkley Books, 1986.

Strauss, Richard H., ed. *Sports Medicine and Physiology.* Philadelphia: W. B. Saunders Company, 1979.

Tarlov, Edward and David D'Costa. *Back Attack.* Boston: Little, Brown and Company, 1985.

Toufexis, A. "The Aching Back." *Time* 14 July 1980: 30–38.

White, Augustus A. *Your Aching Back.* New York: Bantam Books, 1983.

White, A. A. and S. L. Gordon, eds. *Symposium on Idiopathic Low Back Pain.* St. Louis, MO: C. V. Mosby, 1982.

White, A. A. and M. M. Panjabi. "The Clinical Biomechanics of Spine Pain" (Chapter 6). *The Clinical Biomechanics of the Spine.* Philadelphia: J. B. Lippincott, 1978.

Williams, Paul C. *Low Back and Neck Pain.* Springfield, IL: Charles C. Thomas, Publisher, 1974.

---. *The Lumbosacral Spine—Emphasizing Conservative Management.* New York: McGraw-Hill Book Company, 1965.

ABOUT THE AUTHORS

A graduate of Marquette University and the Medical College of Wisconsin, James Wheeler, M.D. is currently an orthopedic surgeon and team physician at the United States Military Academy at West Point, New York.

Author of nearly thirty sports and fitness books, James A. Peterson, Ph.D. is a professor in the Department of Physical Education at the United States Military Academy at West Point, New York.